Believe...

ANGELS DON'T LIE

Believe... Angels Don't Lie

A Heavenly View of God's Plan for Your Well-Being

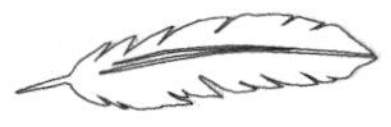

Jeanne Street

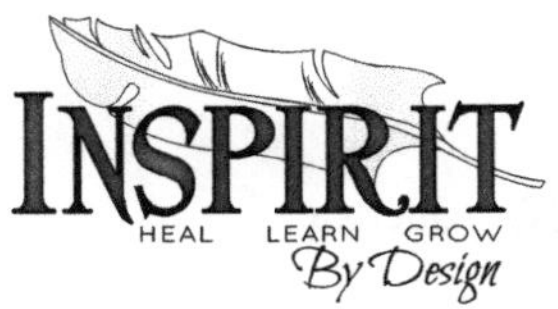

Believe...
Angels Don't Lie

A Heavenly View of God's Plan for Your Well-Being

The information contained within this book by the author is not intended as medical or treatment advice. The intent of the author is to offer information and insight for your
overall spiritual health and well being. The author and publisher assume no responsibility for the misuse, misinterpretations or actions that lead to a particular outcome of a situation or of your life.

Published by: Inspirit by Design, a division of Jeanne Street LLC, New Milford, Connecticut. Cover & interior design and illustrations by: Eileen Portelance, New Milford, CT.

Library of Congress Cataloging-in-Publication Data
Library of Congress Control Number: 2019910426
HARDCOVER ISBN: 978-0-9974666-6-9
PAPERBACK ISBN: 978-0-9974666-7-6
EPUP ISBN: 978-0-9974666-8-3

Second Edition, June 2020
Printed in the United States Of America

To my beloved Brian, for everything you are and for believing me when I told you: Angels don't lie.

Contents

Foreword

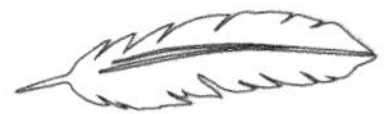

I first met Jeanne in 1985. We were both young, married and pregnant—she with her first child and I with my second. We have been close friends since that very first encounter and have spent many years raising our children and navigating the details of life together. She has been a constant source of love, support, and companionship for me, and I am so grateful for her friendship.

Throughout the years, I have been fortunate to witness Jeanne grow and evolve into the incredible woman she is today. I have always loved her and enjoyed her company, but as she's opened to her spiritual truth, I have come to truly admire who she is, what she does, and her commitment to bringing her best to every interaction she has, for it is evident she believes that each encounter is Divine and each moment is precious.

It has been an honor and a privilege to bear witness to her evolving gifts as a medium and spiritual healer. Through her process of "coming out" and publicly accepting her gifts, I've seen the challenges she faces. The world at large isn't always the most open to or supportive of the spiritual arena. When she began to listen to her calling and speak her truth out loud, she was often met with resistance, doubt, and naysayers who would cause her to question if the messages she was receiving and the gift she had been given were legitimate. After all, she wasn't suddenly saying, "Oh, by the way, I discovered I am incredibly gifted at sewing and I thought you should know," but rather, "I am receiving these messages from the Divine, and I feel like you would benefit from hearing them." That news is a little harder for most people to accept. But message by message, as she began to trust and share, she continued to receive confirmation that her gift was indeed real. She shared messages that there was no way for her to have known; the only explanation was that they were not from her but given through her directly from Divine Source. The more she trusted, the more frequently and clearly the messages came.

I watched as the Divine began to ask more and more of her: *Write a book about the principles we have shown you and that you have used to heal your own life; open a healing studio so that other healers can collaborate and experience practicing healing work together; start a radio show so that you can bring these Divine healing messages beyond your immediate community; start an online learning forum so that people who are grieving and searching for healing, learning, and growing can participate from the comforts of their own home; write a second book.* The requests from the Divine continue and somehow, Jeanne keeps listening to that small, persistent voice. Despite her fears, she does what is asked of her anyway.

I now have the privilege of supporting Jeanne as a scribe in group readings. Oftentimes, attendees are so engrossed in the moment while hearing Jeanne's messages that they have a hard time remembering the details later; this is where my notes provide value. In performing this role, I have witnessed many miracles. I have also been able to collect stories from clients who were so touched they wanted to share their experiences with Jeanne's readers. I'll share three of them here, starting with Joanne's:

> *I came to see Jeanne Street for the first time shortly after the tragic and sudden loss of my husband of thirty-seven years. Our two daughters and I were devastated. His passing sent me reeling. The sadness was crippling. I couldn't imagine my life without him.*
>
> *I knew from my very first meeting with Jeanne that, with her help,*

my broken heart could be mended. The spiritual guidance, support, and loving messages that Jeanne conveyed to me began to ease my pain and set me on a path to healing. I soon realized that I had to rid my mind of the ever-present, fear-based thoughts; I needed to reconnect with God and let love in.

Jeanne's first book, **The Goddess You**, *became my guide. The principles and action steps focused and empowered me. I began to rediscover my relationship with God. I learned to quiet my mind and listen. Prayer, meditation, reiki, yoga, journaling, healing sessions, and readings with Jeanne opened my heart and my eyes to the power of the Divine. Although Tom was no longer by my side in the physical world, he was still very much with me. Through his messages, I found relief. I was not alone, not broken. I had nothing to fear. I needed to be still, forgive, and call on the Divine for the help I needed. Everything was going to be all right.*

I began receiving signs that were miraculous and comforting. It became clear that the bond Tom and I shared in life did not end with his death. One day, the covered dish in which I had often left Tom's dinner shattered in a closed cabinet with no apparent cause. For several weeks, a brilliant scarlet cardinal greeted me with a song each morning when I walked my dogs. Most incredible of all was when I considered the removal of about twenty gangly perennials that were blocking the growth of a small lilac bush in my yard. They were well established, so removing them would be a great deal of work. I reluctantly decided I'd have to live with them. The morning after making that decision, they were gone! I could find no trace of them. My helpful husband was listening. These signs were reflective of Tom in life. With Jeanne's spiritual guidance, I opened my heart to these miracle moments and found both peace and joy in knowing he was still with me.

The insight Jeanne has gained through her own journey, coupled with her gifts of mediumship and healing, are blessings that she so lovingly and graciously shares with others. This book, **Believe...Angels Don't Lie**, *will be a further testament to the power of both God and the Angels, who are always there to help and protect us.*

Jeanne's words will attest to the transformations that the people she has worked with have undergone. I believe hearing stories of miraculous healing and hope will inspire others to shed fear, release grief, and take charge in living the amazing life that God offers.

I am a very different person than I was when I met with Jeanne for the first time. While I am still healing from the trauma of losing Tom, I no longer see myself as a victim. I am a survivor. People deal with grief in many ways, some of which are solitary and self-destructive. I was determined not to take that route. While I will always miss Tom, I am working toward living the life he'd want for me and the life which God intended for all of us. When we face adversity in our lives, we also learn valuable lessons.

I will be forever grateful to Jeanne Street. I know that **Believe... Angels Don't Lie** *will provide inspirational stories of faith, healing and love on every page. If you open your heart to receive, I know that it will change your life.*

—Joanne Reynolds

Joanne's letter is a beautiful testament to the fact we never lose our connection with our loved ones who pass; they have merely transformed from the spiritual body contained in a physical body to a spiritual-only body, no longer contained at all. Joanne also shows us how quickly we can change when we begin to address the fear that governs our thoughts and shift toward love.

Grief is phenomenally powerful. Many of us find that we can be even closer to our loved ones after they pass; indeed, a good deal of healing can take place long after a soul leaves its body. Caitlyn, another of Jeanne's clients, shares her healing story.

I am a wife, sister, daughter, and mother of two young children. I have experienced grief in my life, but never to the extent I felt in September of 2017. A week after his seventy-first birthday, my dad passed away. I've always believed in God, Heaven, and Angels. I asked my dad in his final days if he was going to become an Angel. With labored breath, he said, "I don't want to talk about that." Then I asked if he wanted me to pray with him. He nodded, so we held hands and prayed together. I requested that God let him know how much he was loved, take his pain away, let him know we would all be okay if he had to leave us, and to show him beautiful healing light. That night, I left my dad's bedside and glanced back for one more good-bye as he blew me a kiss. This was the last time I saw my father alive.

The lyrics of a song I listened to after his passing about wanting to make a father proud touched me deeply. When he was alive, he told me he was proud of me. He told me I was beautiful. He told me I was talented. I never listened; I brushed off his compliments, thinking he just said it because that's what dads are supposed to say. I wish it hadn't taken his death for me to believe him. But in the same breath, I am thankful to have received the Divine message of his pride in me. And that wouldn't have been possible without Jeanne.

I have always been intrigued by spiritual mediums, and when I saw a local coffee shop was hosting a group reading, I read about Jeanne and immediately purchased my ticket. I was afraid to admit how desperately I wanted to hear from my dad. I told myself it would be neat to hear others connect with loved ones, and I believed that if no one came through for me, that would be okay. When I arrived that night, I could feel something special in the air. Jeanne came to me and said there was a man there who wanted to talk to me and was telling me not to leave. I knew it was my dad right away. It shocked me that he was telling her to not let me leave, because I had been considering it. I had left my baby, whom I always put to sleep, at home for bedtime. When I had sat down, I'd thought to myself, ***If this is getting to be too long and she passes by me without any Angel messages, I may have to sneak out to get home to the baby.***

While I wasn't looking for "proof," Jeanne had it, and many more points that confirmed to me my dad was there talking to her, like how he was standing up and pointing to his legs saying how great he felt. He had been in pain and unable to walk for a few years before he passed—but Jeanne had no way of knowing that.

The biggest message was when she told me he was beaming with pride for me. Hearing this reminded me of all the things he had said when he was alive that I didn't take time to listen to. Hearing through Jeanne that he's proud of me opened my heart in a way I didn't know could be opened. The lesson I learned and continue to learn from Jeanne through her presence and her writing is that even though I didn't appreciate my father's words while he was here, I can find a new appreciation through her Divine message from him.

When my dad passed away, my grief felt like cement poured into my chest. It would hit me hard at random times and knock the wind out of me. But there is a reason that clichés like "It feels like a weight was lifted" exist. I know this to be true because that's the feeling I experienced after hearing from my father through Jeanne. My life shifted, and my grief decreased because I became open to messages from Heaven. That night changed my life, and I hope that by reading my story and the other messages in this book, others can find comfort in truly believing that our loved ones are never far from us. God placed people like Jeanne on Earth to show us the truth in this.

— Caitlyn Doenges

The grief we experience from the loss of a loved one can sometimes feel like we are underwater with a rock on top of us, making it so hard to go on with our own lives. Caitlyn's story is an example of how hearing a message from our loved one after they pass can lift that weight. We discover that we have not ended our relationships with the death of our loved ones' bodies. To the contrary, our departed loved ones are happy and free, and they want us to continue living the life we are meant to live.

Mediums don't only work with death; they also work with healing. In the following, Kathy tells her story of confusion and fear surrounding her daughter's health, which transforms to one of clarity and hope after Jeanne helped her connect to her loved ones on the other side who were able to offer her messages of love and reassurance. In Kathy's words:

I first met Jeanne at Sassy Shoe, a neighborhood shop that she owned and operated in town. At the time, I was working at a local nonprofit, organizing community impact programs and principally coordinating the collection and distribution of clothing and school supplies to local children in need. Jeanne kindly hosted a fundraiser at her store to promote awareness and financial services for our program, and later donated dozens of children's shoes to the charity after the store's closing.

Several years passed, and I unexpectedly ran into Jeanne in town. She immediately sensed that I was struggling. My daughter had fallen ill and was silently suffering from a chronic, undiagnosed illness. I had left my work at the nonprofit to care for her, and she and I were both seeking answers and peace that medical doctors were unable to provide us. Jeanne immediately insisted that we visit her home the following day so that she could perform her healing techniques on my daughter. Our visit was overwhelmingly emotional, but through it all, Jeanne was gentle, loving, patient, and knowledgeable. We left with a profound sense of peace and hope for a future diagnosis, which we ultimately received from doctors less than a month after visiting with her.

When Jeanne opened her studio, I immediately began to follow her journey on social media, intrigued and fascinated by her incredible love and wisdom of Angels and God. I was raised in a Catholic home, inherited a strong appreciation for Angels from my late mother, felt an incredible connection to God through prayer, and was always looking for signs from loved ones who had passed. My girlfriend and I attended a private reading at Jeanne's lovely, tranquil studio, and three of my dear loved ones came through with beautiful messages of hope and faith. My nephew passed away as a young adult after a debilitating ailment slowly deteriorated his physical and mental health. When he, my mother, and grandmother came through in the reading, I expressed concern about whether the cause of his death could have been hereditary, thinking of the possible connection to my daughter. He assured me that his illness had actually been a viral infection. My mother and grandmother reassured me about my other concerns and grievances.

Since having such powerful and positive experiences with Jeanne, I faithfully tune in to her Facebook Live angel card readings as well as her **Angels Don't Lie** *radio show (transitioned into a podcast), which she hosts weekly. I truly look forward to these sessions and thoroughly enjoy her inspirational messages and wellness insights. Jeanne has sincerely enriched my life, and I am forever grateful for her knowledge, philosophy, energy, and goodness.*

— *Kathy Thomas*

Despite this praise, Jeanne remains humble. She seems to be in utter awe and honor of the messages that the Divine conveys through her to loved ones in need. She continues to listen and follow the guidance she is given from the Divine and willingly shares the loving, healing, and uplifting messages that she receives. She is keenly aware that the messages are Divine truth and she is the vessel.

Over the past three decades, witnessing Jeanne's personal transformation take place has brought so much joy to my life. And I am pleased to continue watching her inspire others shift their life's path in profound ways. Again and again, Jeanne shows up to perform the tasks the Divine asks of her. She plainly states that when Spirit speaks, she is listening and that Angels don't lie!

— *Colleen Fairchild*

Introduction

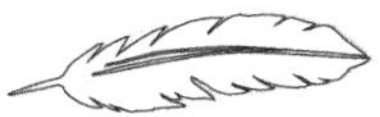

I have always been an energetically sensitive gal, a Divine truth seeker who is deeply inquisitive about issues of mystical wisdom. I've had the *knowing*, the undeniable truth and wisdom that flows from the Divine and through my being for as long as I can remember.

And, like so many of us, I denied my personal truth out of fear.

Believe you are love. All of us originated from the Source, which is Divine love. Our need to connect and fill ourselves with love is the reason we find ourselves drawn to books such as the one you are now holding in your hands. This need to connect is what pulls us toward the people, places, and things that return our investment of time and energy by feeding our beautiful souls with love and brightening the light within us.

Energy Exchange

We are energy; we give energy and we receive energy. We search for guidance and help that will support, guide, and comfort us as we come to a deeper understanding of our experiences. Life is uniquely challenging for each of us. We are wounded, we suffer, and we carry pain within our being that comes in peaks and valleys. Our mind chatters away from thought to thought to avoid this. Then, a combination of fear and ego that I call *Shmego* shows up to challenge or take away our happiness. Our Shmego guy tests our joy and, if we do not pass this test, leaves us feeling isolated and alone.

Yet at other times, we are able to celebrate our joys and successes. We are able to live in the moment. We can even look at diversity head on with love, strength and compassion, and shine confidently as the unique beings that we are.

We all have versions of these highs and lows. We also commonly have feelings arise such as anxiety, depression, shame, and fear of being judged. At times we give these energies out to others, sometimes without realizing we are doing so.

About This Book

We are magical souls capable of healing our greatest source of pain with angelic guidance. I have learned something on this spiritual journey of mine, something that has saved me from inner turmoil and denying who I am: the art of maintaining a spiritual connection with Divine love and higher power, God. Now relax and breathe, this is not about religion! I call my higher power *God*; sometimes I even replace it with *Divine*, *Source,* or *Spirit.* You are free to call your higher power whatever feels right to you.

In this book, I share insightful and intimate details from some of my clients' readings, healing sessions, miraculous healings, and heavenly messages. These are intended to assist you in freeing yourself from energy that no longer serves you, while healing your pain and suffering. You too can connect to the Divine realm, along with the Angels and celestial beings within it, to live your purpose-filled and meaningful life.

Come along with me on this heavenly, insightful journey. I will showcase what it's like to live life spiritually and soulfully connected. I will also illuminate how to discover your God-given gifts within. This will allow you to invite Divine love in and dramatically shift your life.

Throughout this book, I offer you a chance to delve deeper into learning, healing, and growing with the help of exercises, including guided meditations, general journal suggestions, and specific journal prompts. I share insights from client readings and examples from my own life that show how Divine messages can both guide and heal fear, grief, trauma, and painful life circumstances. You will witness miracles within these experiences. Please note that clients' names have been changed to honor and protect their privacy.

This book gives a celestial view of how God's heavenly Angels want to be your guide in healing. They want to raise consciousness—both your individual consciousness and that of the collective. Your personal life will shift as you become more open to receiving and as you choose to accept Divine love. You will find that believing in and connecting to the Angels increases your energy; your thoughts will rise from a lower, fear-based vibration to a higher, love-based vibration. What once seemed impossible will feel full of ease.

Following, I have included a glossary of words and definitions that I will be using in this book.

Believe Angels Don't Lie Glossary

The Twelve Goddess Principles. The twelve Goddess principles are meant as tools to achieve connection to our highest selves. (I explain them in much greater detail in my first book, *The Goddess You.*)

1. ***Quieting the Mind:*** We calm our brain chatter by learning how to shift our fear-based thoughts over to love-based thoughts.

2. ***Self-Love:*** We mirror to the world what we think and feel about ourselves, and we receive that same energy back into our lives. If we want more love to come in, we must learn to love ourselves!

3. ***Changing Your Reactions:*** Silence is golden; we can learn a lot about ourselves when we quiet our inner and outer chatter. The real power we have comes from practicing compassion.

4. ***Energy Basics:*** Energy can get stuck and build up, causing blocks within our life. This can make day-to-day life a challenge. Cleaning

your energy up is how you discern the difference between your energy and someone else's.

5. ***Healing the Block:*** Our intent to heal and release our pain requires the actions of practicing faith, forgiveness, and surrender.

6. ***Let It Go:*** Sharing our stories and replaying past memories over and over causes them to build walls within our being, blocking love from filling us. Removing our story, brick by brick, is how we can align with our Soul Self.

7. ***Chakra Basics:*** Each chakra point in our body is a pathway for energy to enter. They bring us into closer connection with God and allow for us to receive and emit love. Clearing these points with meditation and energy work brings forth another level of healing.

8. ***Healthy, Wealthy, and Wise:*** Knowing our body's energy and vibrational rate helps us to know what our body, mind, and soul need to maintain our highest, healthiest energy level.

9. ***Keep Calm:*** Entering our crazy stress states is never a good feeling. Finding our calm in the challenging times is important for the well-being of our mind, body, and soul.

10. ***Help, I've Lost My Balance:*** Our balance comes from layering the twelve principles together. Knowing how to get our energy back in alignment is our newfound survival tool!

11. ***Mind, Body, and Spirit:*** Living in alignment with our Soul Self will shift our energy, raise our vibration, and open the channels to receive Spirit's guidance through our intuition.

12. ***Intuitive, Gifted You:*** Faith in God and in ourselves is the proven tool to achieve our personal enlightened state of living. Soul alignment is the new sexy!

Cycle Breathing. This type of breath requires you to breathe in through your nose and out through your mouth. Follow your breath on the inhalation, holding it within your belly before slowly exhaling it out of your mouth. You will need to do this in several exercises throughout the book; try it now and see how it goes!

Divine Masculine. Our connection to healthy, non-fear-based ego and earth-based logic. Every soul has a Divine masculine side, regardless of gender.

Divine Feminine. The flow of spirituality and love, which are our connection to God. Every soul has a Divine feminine side, regardless of gender.

God. Also called Source, Spirit, or the Divine. In this book the word *God* refers to the higher power, or the energy, that we tap into which is beyond us and that represents where we originate. Though I reference Christianity and Christian concepts frequently in this book, the God that I am writing about is not specifically Christian; rather, Christianity just provides a framework to use when we describe Him. In fact, one great synonym for God is *Love*!

Soul Self. Also known as enlightenment, the authentic self, and/or the Goddess self, the Soul Self is the highest version of you. This represents the balance of the Divine feminine and Divine masculine. It is what illuminates our path, the truth of who we are, and what we have come here to accomplish.

Goddess Truths. Your Goddess truths are the unique, Divine truths of who you are and why you are here.

Shmego. As noted earlier, Shmego is the name I have given ego when it has been taken over by fear. This energy is very dangerous and can hijack your life.

Fear Addiction. To have a fear addiction is to be dependent on thoughts that are fear-based rather than love-based.

"You Work." When I refer to the "you work," I refer to the time you spend on your well-being, learning, healing, growing, and evolving.

Sacred Space. This is the physical and energetic space in which you do your "you work" to heal, learn, and grow. Sacred space can be manifested outwardly, as a room or temple, or inwardly, as the space within your being in which you hold prayers for others, offer forgiveness, or let go of past pains.

Altar. An altar is a space where you place religious or other significant items that are dedicated to your spiritual growth.

Sensitive Soul. A *sensitive soul* is blessed with the gift of compassion and is commonly called a highly sensitive person (HSP). Their senses of feeling and emotion are heightened, meaning they receive energy through one or more senses when triggered by the people or animals around them. Unlike an empath, a sensitive soul experiences these interactions purely on the outside of their body.

Empath. An empath is a person who can physically tune in to the emotional energy of a person or an animal. Their intuition, emotions, and feelings are heightened. This gift also comes with one or more heightened senses that, unlike a sensitive soul's, are felt not only externally but also internally; the energy flows inside the body, and they physically experience the feelings of another.

"Nancy Drew it." To "Nancy Drew it" means to become a detective of how, what, and why our senses are being activated. In turn, this helps us distinguish how Spirit is guiding us.

Chakras. The chakras are energy centers located in and around the physical body. They are points of connection for Divine love to flow.

Christ Points. The Christ points are Divine energy centers located in the soles of your feet and palms of your hands.

Karma. Borrowing from Eastern philosophy, karma is the result of misdeeds. It is the energy that all souls carry with them until the wrong deed is healed and transformed into love.

On Journaling

To achieve the intent of this book, you'll have to do the "you work" by journaling, which will help you organize your thoughts. You will find that there is truth in the words you write; there are answers to the questions you are pondering. Taking these actions will serve your soul. This is proven: science has shown that when we write in a journal, our minds enter a meditative state, which I agree creates an open space for personal discovery.

Keep your journal near you while you read, as well as a dedicated pen or pencil so you are ready to go whenever you need to start writing. This is your tool for conversing with your Soul Self and the Divine realm! If you want to go even deeper, I've created additional resources that will continue to support you on your journey of healing and working with the Angels. You can find these at ***believeangels.com***.

There are two universal truths that the Angels shared with me which are worth mentioning now. The first truth is that our souls are infinite, meaning we are here on this earthly plane and we are with God. We are expansive beings, if we so choose, we can connect to our Soul Self and live a joyful life. Since we are all infinite, our departed loved ones are therefore always with us—just without physical form. The second truth is that we all want to be loved and validated. Through my experience channeling readings for clients, I have been shown that their departed loved ones and their team of Angels are in agreement that we are all in need of a love intervention.

My Own Fear Addiction

In my twenties and thirties, I actually thought that people who talked about Angels were a little freaky. It's true—really! Even though I had departed souls visiting my room when I was a child, I never fully understood that seeing those souls was a gift. I thought everyone experienced energy the same way I did. It took some doing, but the Angels finally got my attention and I learned how to honor and work with this special gift. (If you want to know more about my journey and how you can better know your own gifts, you can read more about them in my book *The Goddess You*.)

The Angels told me that my aversion toward Angel communicators was born out of my fear addiction. Essentially, I was living in denial—denial not only of admitting and sharing my gift, but also denial of God. I never fully grasped that by denying the existence of my gift and His Angels, I was in turn denying God. They revealed that God is all of Heaven and Earth and that Angels are His Divine beings. In believing any soul is separate from God, we deny Him.

If you had told me back then, I would never have believed that I, a shy Catholic girl who denied the existence of Angels, would someday be conversing with these celestial beings on matters of great importance for both myself and others. As the saying goes, "You live and you learn!" Now, years later, I am conversing with the Angels as I write a book entitled *Believe... Angels Don't Lie*!

I mean, seriously!

Why Journey Through Pain?

I assure you that the journey to heal your pain and open your communication to the Angels is well worth your time and effort. Now that I am on the other side of my fear addiction, I am able to fully embrace the woo-woo, crunchy, yoga enthusiast, New-Agey, God-loving side of myself, and I can honestly state it was the best decision I have ever made! And, my friend, it is my sincere hope that connecting to the Angels and embracing your truths, even those freaky things about yourself, will lead you to living your best life in union with your Soul Self.

Since braving the shadows of fear and the illusion that I was not enough, I've experienced moments that have humbled me and blessed my life. In readings and healing sessions, I've channeled Jesus, Holy Mother Mary, and the Holy Spirit. I have connected clients to their departed loved ones and helped them to release and heal grief that had morphed into physical illness. I have also had the privilege of sharing Divine messages and guidance on my weekly Podcast and Facebook Live show, also called *Angels Don't Lie*.

We are here on this Earth for a short time, and no matter how much you may deny it, run or hide: there you are. It's scary, a little funny, and yet oh-so-true!

The Angels say that life is a beautiful privilege meant to be cherished and lived well, even with the bumps and turns in the road. My dear friend, now is your time to start loving yourself and living your best life by going through the steps that I've mapped out for you in this book.

Meet me on the next page, and I'll introduce you to the Angels!

Blessings,

xx Jeanne

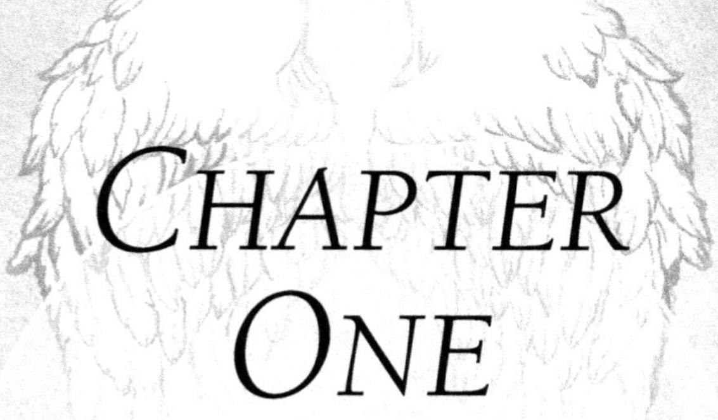

Chapter One

CHAPTER ONE

ANGELS

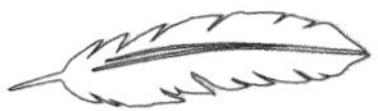

"For He will command His angels concerning you to guard you in all your ways. On their hands they will bear you up, lest you strike your foot against a stone."

— *PSALM 91:11–12 ESV*

When talking about Angels, I like to tell my clients and peeps that Angels have our backs day in and day out. Especially so when we are open to receiving their help by inviting them into our life.

We are souls who have been incarnated in human form. In this form, our main focus is to remember love. Being human means that you and I are equally flawed, meaning that we each have our own unique qualities, some of which we may believe are flaws. Our flaws can be the call to grow and change an old pattern or belief. Yet we are nevertheless still beautiful souls. In being flawed, we have the opportunity to learn many lessons through our human experience. Though some experiences are harder to process than others, great blessings come with each lesson learned—yet when those experiential lessons become uncomfortable, our energy can instantly plummet without our conscious permission.

In a world full of fear, claiming responsibility for our personal and collective consciousness is of great importance. When we rise to the occasion by choosing love over that which no longer serves us, we must first address our connection to Source. We have to heal our experiences, not just try to forget them. We are in a time and place where it seems almost normal to walk away from painful memories and cut people out of our lives before understanding and healing the reason we experienced what we did. We've become a throwaway society on so many levels that it's scary.

What I have come to know and fully trust is that when I am sharing Spirit's messages with either a single client, a small group, a large audience, over video or in writing, a collective healing occurs. I have witnessed, through prayer, connection to Divine Source and Spirit's guiding messages, that in order for us to be spiritually whole, we have to put the time and effort into working on our relationship with God and with our higher self.

Finding Our Faith

When we feel stuck in life, unable to see a light at the end of our tunnel of despair, it's time for a lifeline of hope to come in and help us to rise above our situation. We don't feel depleted and stuck in our life because we lack talent or worth; it's always been about Divine timing. Our joy is determined by several factors, like where we are in learning a lesson and whether we have released the energy that binds us to this time and place. It's also related to our level of faith. On a scale of one to ten, how much faith do you have?

It is commonplace for us to become so busy with family, friends, work, and our to-do lists that we forget to stop and take a breath of air. It's also pretty common for us to try and negotiate with God rather than trust the process and allow ourselves the experience of our "now." It's not a common practice to say a prayer asking for angelic guidance. Sometimes I even forget to call on them!

But doing this is dangerous, because when we put our wants above all else, we lose focus on what's real and where love is available to us. We can shift this by regularly committing to doing our "you work." Doing our "you work" is the most necessary component in reaching our desired outcome because it forces us to focus on love rather than lack.

Braedyn's story, which follows, exemplifies what happens when we trust the process. It shows the miracles that can occur when we are connected to God, surrendering our need to control, and practicing full faith.

The moment I met baby Braedyn is one I will keep forever in my heart. He was six months old. He had been diagnosed in utero with clubfoot (a diagnosis that was later retracted) and a rare brain disorder called lissencephaly, also known as "smooth brain."

His parents, Katie and Jonathan, had experienced many challenges and emotions through their struggles with fertility before conceiving Braedyn. They faced many more during the pregnancy, the delivery, and following his birth. Unsure of the outcome, both their spirits and their faith had plummeted. It seemed every time they turned a corner, they were met with more worries and little hope for his survival. By the time their infant son was released from the hospital, hospice care was already in place. His parents tiptoed emotionally through each moment, wondering if it may be his last.

I knew about this through my daughter, Lauren, who is friends with Katie. I had also been following the family's journey on Facebook and had been sending distant healing and prayers to them. Katie knew that I was a healer and, once Braedyn was born, she decided to seek out different types of holistic care. She reached out to me, asking if I could work with babies, and we set up our first session for the following week.

Before every session, I open for an *Angel call*—a form of meditation where I am transported to a celestial plane. During the time in this plane, the energy of God is shared through Jesus or other ascended masters, along with my team of Angels. They will impress upon me how each reading or healing session will flow. I will also be guided as to what tools or methods to use in the upcoming session.

As I was preparing for Braedyn's first session, I received the message that the session would be directed at reinstilling faith. When Katie walked into the studio with Braedyn, God's love filled my being. As I began, I held my hands over Braedyn's heart, and an instant soul connection was made. I then moved from focusing on Braedyn's health issues to focusing on Katie's current state of being. I was guided by the Angels to proceed in a direct and slow manner to deliver messages to Katie. A departed loved one came through with reassurance and supportive love for their family. I was impressed with the image of the number *six* along with the message that there were more souls waiting to come into their family if they ever decided to have more children. I could feel Katie's relief in my body as her departed loved one shared how Braedyn would surprise the medical doctors with his strength. I also was impressed with the sense that all would be well, and though they would experience setbacks, Braedyn would develop beyond expectations. I knew that this meant there would be a miracle moment, and we would see it when the timing was right.

In subsequent sessions with Braedyn, I was guided to work more with crystals and sound healing. After one session where I was guided to make a large circle of amethyst crystals around his body, the Angels impressed an image within my mind of a baby blanket with tiny chips of amethyst sewn into it. The vision was as clear as a photograph. I shared what I'd seen with my daughter, Lauren, and asked her if she would help me create this blanket for Braedyn. Being an experienced mother of four and foster mother to fourteen, I instinctively knew that the main part of the blanket needed to house the crystals while an outer cover could be taken off for washing. Lauren and I joined forces, united in love, to create this vision. The end product was truly a labor of love. When Braedyn and Katie arrived for our next session, I placed the blanket on the healing table. When Katie put him down on the blanket, the smile on his face was all I needed to know that he felt the Divine love and healing being offered from his new comfort blanket.

The day came for a miracle to be revealed. Up to this point, Spirit hadn't shown me Braedyn as a young man. In my pre-session Angel call, Jesus showed me a singing bowl being played over Braedyn's head, and I knew that the vibrational music waves would open a higher level of healing for him. I shared this with Katie when she came for the session. As I played the rose quartz singing bowl, Braedyn's face lit up with joy. His whole body absorbed the energy as Spirit sent more messages for Katie. I shared how Jesus had shown me Braedyn as an adolescent. Since his body was going through many changes, I saw that he could possibly need surgery or a GI tube from other issues related to his inverted intestines. The Angels also said that there were going to be visible, miraculous changes in his next MRI. I always offer each client follow-up instructions to aid their healing journey, and after this particular session, I suggested that Katie download singing bowl music for Braedyn.

About a week later, I received word from Katie that Braedyn had been rediagnosed. Based on genetic and brain testing, Braedyn's diagnosis had changed from lissencephaly, which comes with a life expectancy cap, to septo-optic dysplasia, which does not. She explained how, though this neurological disorder would still bring developmental delays, the limits of what Braedyn could or couldn't do were no longer defined.

A miracle can only be revealed when we are ready to receive it. Being ready does not happen by forcing an outcome or denying love, rather it comes from participating in our own healing by doing our "you work."

Katie's restoration of faith was the "you work" she needed to do. Her willingness to participate in her healing and make changes following the Angels' guidance was crucial to me receiving the image of Braedyn as a young man. And there was an immediate payoff, because that was the moment when Katie's hope and faith returned. Had Katie not been open and ready to receive Divine love through angelic messages, this miracle moment would not have happened. If we are not open to receiving God's love, the Angels cannot offer us guidance. It is a matter of free will; it's up to us to choose love or deny it.

Finding Joy in the Process

"See, I am sending an angel ahead of you to guard you along the way and to bring you to the place I have prepared."

— *EXODUS 23:20 NIV*

The truth is that we are never fully complete in our healing work. This life that we have been gifted is a true adventure and we are here to experience, evolve, and emerge out of fear and into love's embrace.

But how can we experience joy when we are always either working on healing or still in pain?

I wondered this myself, so I did what I do best: I sat down on my meditation pillow to talk with God and the Angels. The answer that came was to look back on the life I've created for myself by following the twelve Goddess principles.

This view showed me that by connecting with and channeling Spirit for the people who come my way, I am not only witnessing profound truths and healing for my clients, but they are also healing truths for my soul. I can experience joy while this healing is taking place because the process of healing itself becomes joyful.

By living in alignment with my Goddess truth, I've experienced how expressing love through the action of my gifts helps ignite others to use their gifts as well. The same is true for each of us. When we share our Goddess truths by expressing our gifts and talents, we help others in turn. When we choose to live in alignment and express our soul's truths as spiritual beings, we provide an example for others on how living a soul-aligned life can bring forth love, passion, and joy.

The Angels often impress the truth that we are not yet fully aware of the profound impact we have on others' lives. The healing that comes when a message is delivered is an undeniable force of Divine love at work. I have witnessed immense healing take place when clients hear from their loved ones who are no longer living in the physical world. This healing can alter clients' paths profoundly, allowing them to make the necessary changes to improve their life's circumstances. I have also experienced personal healing from past events and traumas just from delivering these messages to others. I feel an emotional connection to both my clients and their loved ones in Heaven. It is a mystical bond that connects through time and space.

The Role of Fear

As souls in human form, we were created to feel emotions as a way to receive and express love. Unfortunately, many painful experiences cause a separation from love, and fear moves in to take its place.

Fear is a feeling, an emotion, and an action. Fear can be felt internally as well as delivered to others. Fear tells us lies to keep us victims to the circumstances of our lives.

But fear doesn't need to stop us from having our Divine conversation. My favorite part of talking with God and his team of celestial beings is that I get to be my authentic self. I can speak candidly to Spirit just as I would a friend; no filter, just plain ol' me. We can show up real, broken, afraid, worried or angry, and we are accepted just as we are! I keep my conversations real, swear at times, and use a firm voice when necessary in order get an important point across. In that conversation, we get to drop our fear at the door, because as celestial beings of Divine love, Angels will never judge us or our choices. Their job is beautiful and simple: they get to gently guide and illuminate our path.

The ultimate goal is for you to find your soul's truth by learning and growing through your own Goddess truth. This brings the soul into alignment, which some call *enlightenment*.

What I have learned from the Angels is that every soul is connected to God, but not everyone chooses to open to and live within that connection. When we are connected to our higher self, our lives flow with ease. The connection to our Soul Self is a vertical and boundless light energy. You can see it as a cord of energy that connects from the crown of your head to your Soul Self in Heaven. This energy cord gets blocked or shut off over time with the debris left over from life's experiences. Your goal to living your life in alignment, being on your soul's path, and living your purpose is to strengthen the connection flowing through this Divine cord.

"The soul is placed in the body like a rough diamond and must be polished, or the luster of it will never appear."

— *DANIEL DEFOE*

Exercise

When you feel doubt, when you're unsure of something you're feeling, or when you're pondering the truth of something you're reading, take a moment to do the following core color meditation exercise to align with your Soul Self. The Angels guided me to develop this powerful tool to help guide us back into faith. It works with everything, from relationships to foods, medication, readings, writing, and more!

Core Color Meditation:

Begin by breathing and setting your intention to connect to your Soul Self. Take a moment to breathe in and out several times while sitting upright with your feet planted firmly on the ground.

With an inhalation, bring your attention to the soles of your feet. The soles of your feet connect you to the here and now, and to your place on Earth. Cycle your breath several times until you feel the energy or sensation begin to move in your feet.

Now bring your attention to the crown of your head. The crown is your connection to the flow of Divine love and truth. Breathe in and out as you invite the crown to open. You may feel goose bumps or feel your torso sway as the energy begins to flow.

Move your awareness to the center of your chest, your heart center. This is the seat of your soul, where you and God connect. As you bring your breath into your heart center, you will feel expansive, loved, and safe.

As you continue to breathe into your heart center, imagine your breath connecting with a color. This color will emerge as you breathe; it may have been your favorite color your entire life, or one you recall from your childhood. This is your soul's core color.

There is no right or wrong color, as only you know your core color. Don't stress if you are unable to connect with your color right away; just pick a color and move on. With practice your confidence will grow, sparking your clear intuitive connection to your core color.

After you've connected with your color for a while, bring your focus back to the crown of your head and invite the Divine energy from above to flow inward and down past your eyes, through your throat and along the length of your spine. Feel it move past your hips, down your legs, and into your feet. Then bring your awareness back to the center of your chest, your heart center, and notice the two energies begin to merge. Your core color begins to glow more brightly and, with each breath in, this energy flows throughout your body.

Invite the energy to encircle your body as a shimmering sphere of love that embraces your entire being. This is your soul's truth merged with God surrounding you, supporting you, protecting you. Stay here for as long as you like.

In this meditative state, you can find answers and truths and know what is serving you or what is not. Surrounded by this color sphere, connect with whatever it is that you doubt and notice if it is outside your energy sphere or within. If it is within, it serves you. If it appears to you outside of the sphere, you can take a moment to connect to it with your breath, inviting it into your sphere. Notice whether it comes in naturally.

If you first see the item you are questioning within your sphere, this is a clear yes. If it comes in when invited, you have the option to bring it into your life. If it stubbornly remains outside the sphere, it either doesn't serve you at all or it may not be the right time. If this happens, wait a few days and try the exercise again to see if anything changes.

Journal Prompts:

After completing the core color meditation, use the following prompts to write about your experience in your journal:

- How do you feel this energy within your body?
- How does it feel when the item is outside the sphere?
- How does it feel when you move the item into your sphere?

- Where in your body do you feel the energy?
- Does your sphere have moments where it weakens or dulls, or do you see a break in its surface?

Write any additional findings and questions you have.

This exercise will guide you through knowing what serves you and what does not. You can repeat it time and time again to help you discern what is serving you and what is not.

Angels, God, and Sacred Space

Let me tell you more about my dear Angels, how I got to know them and how you, too, can get to know them on a profound and personal level.

The Angels who speak to me are not one singular being but rather a communion of Heavenly-Beings made up of God's energy. This energy emits a pulse which feels like a vibration. Of course, whether we connect to this pulse or not is up to us; free will is always at play here, and our soul's journey as we learn, grow, and evolve are the keys that can either open the door or keep it locked up tight. Our intent is the guidepost; we must have clear intention paired with faith and prayer for our intuition to open fully.

Setting an intention is a deliberate choice. It's a decision that we make. Without a clear intention to connect to God, we are open to receive lower vibrational energy. Lower vibrational energy consists of negative, fearful, dark, or even evil energy. Your intuitive sense, or the sixth sense as some call it, is the conduit for connecting to this energy or picking it up. Your interpretations of the energy can be witnessed through one or sometimes all of the senses. Every soul is born with the ability to connect their senses to the Divine in one way or another. Your senses are also how you will interpret and express the gifts and talents that are unique to you, as well as to every living soul.

One of the important lessons the Angels taught me early on was the need for setting sacred space. As noted earlier, sacred space is where you go to do your "you work," be it a physical place or an internal space.

In order for the Divine to work with you and through you, in order for the Angels and Divine love to be present in your life, you must first establish sacred space. The Angels say setting sacred space is similar to a contract. You set the intention of holding love and compassion for both yourself and for everyone else, with no exceptions. Only then can you agree to do the "you work" and hold yourself at a higher Divine standard of thinking and being. There, fearful thoughts have no value, and love is therefore amplified.

Sacred space can be used in situations of distress, such as in a troubled relationship. Let's take my client Carrie as an example. Carrie came to me for a reading to connect with her deceased father. As soon as I grabbed my journal to scribe impressions, Spirit flooded me with the sense of unease that comes with a drama-filled relationship. In my mind's eye I saw a tornado, which is my sign for drama. I also saw a bull, which signals that someone is bullying or forcing their energy and thoughts on another. I asked Carrie whether she was involved in a relationship that was causing her stress. She looked up with tears streaming down her face and nodded her head. As she did so, Carrie's father came forward out of the veil and pointed to Carrie's chest, impressing in me a heaviness which is my sign for grief. I told Carrie that her father was standing by her side and that he was worried about the grief she was holding on to and carrying with her. Her father then spoke about the troubled relationship that was burdening his daughter and causing her grief over his departure to be amplified. Carrie confirmed that a woman she was working with, one whom she considered a friend, was forcing her opinions, thoughts, and energy onto Carrie. Spirit impressed within my mind the vision of a snake with its tongue out, which for me represents verbal abuse. Carrie said that her friend was using slander and monetary manipulation to control Carrie and the work she was doing.

Carrie's father held his hand on her shoulder to show he was supporting his daughter and spoke with the same gentle tone he had in life. His advice was for Carrie to stop giving her energy away and instead to pull it back and direct it within, toward self-love. He also reminded her that when she chooses love over fear, she will be set free of the controlling energy from this painful relationship. Spirit led me to guide Carrie through creating sacred space for her friend and teach Carrie how to hold her friend in a place of love instead of a place of fear. As it turned out, this was the perfect pathway for healing this situation.

Carrie left our session with the tools she needed to strengthen and heal the way she viewed herself and her friend. This, accompanied by her father's loving messages, eased and lifted her grief.

The Work of Angels

Angels don't always appear in groups: they can appear in singular form as well. No matter how they arrive, their job is to gently guide and support us without interfering with our free will. They can show or reveal themselves to us by taking on an energetic form or flowing in the energy of light. Depending on the person, situation, and circumstance, the Angels will choose the highest and best way to reveal themselves to us. They will never come to instill fear or harm or to influence us negatively. The job of Angels is to serve God, not man, and they do so with Divine, holy love. Like other Divine beings of God's love such as archangels, saints, and ascended masters, Angels gently guide and support us, the ones God loves so much that He calls us His children.

Most of us begin to forget God and Divine love in our young lives, around four to six years of age. We are influenced by others, and the conditioning from the adults in our lives molds our young minds with a new, censored, fearful thought pattern. Once fear enters our thoughts, we then spend the rest of our life questioning God, trying to remember Him, outright denying Him or we can choose to do our "you work" and regain our alignment with God.

Children have perfect memories of God. Ask any toddler who is able to speak and you will hear how they know God and remember Heaven. When my granddaughter Riley was four, she told me how she remembered God. One warm summer day while sitting by our pool, Riley said innocently, sweetly, and entirely out of the blue, "Mom, Mom, when I was in Heaven with God, I was in line to come into Mommy's tummy after Maisy [her younger sister], but I wanted to be first so I pushed her out of the way." I smiled and, with tears of love in my eyes, asked her, "Oh, Riley, what did Maisy do when you pushed her out of the way?" Shrugging her shoulders, Riley replied matter-of-factly, "She cried like she always does!" And that was that; Riley went right back to swimming as if nothing else in the world mattered.

Since that day, Riley has shared several heartwarming moments like this with us. She even brought a message to me from my friends Jodi and Suzy, who had both passed away. The fact that Riley hardly knew Jodi and had never heard of or met my old high-school friend Suzy didn't stop the loving messages from coming through. Riley said, "Mom, Mom, remember your friend with the hair like Kari's? [My cousin and BFF, Kari, has blonde hair similar to Jodi's.] She's saying hello with big purple wings, and her friend that you know with the dark hair is with her. You went to school with her, and she has blue wings. They are dancing and waving at you!" I just about fell over! I had no doubt that Jodi would visit me; I was honored to be by her side and holding her hand on the day she passed from breast cancer. But when she brought Suzy with her I was amazed: we had not spoken in over thirty years.

Most every religion speaks of Angels, spirit beings or devas as God's messengers. Archangels are also God's messengers. They are celestial beings of light, similar to Angels; the only difference is that in the hierarchy of Angels, they are the highest form, closest to God. Archangels are distinctive in their energy, and it is their nature to impart God's will.

We can begin to invite Angels into our lives at any time. Through our intention, prayer, and faith, the Angels can offer loving, gentle support.

Exercise

Practicing this exercise helped open my eyes and life with the Angels. I invite you to try this lovely Angel ceremony as an experiment for yourself. You can choose to start on any given day and continue practicing the ceremony for seven consecutive days. Be sure to journal your mood, feelings, and experience daily, as you will find it helpful to reflect back on your observations.

Angel Ceremony:

Begin by setting a physical altar and holding intention in your internal sacred space where your Angel ceremony will convene for one week. Choose someplace quiet, where you can meditate and reflect. Your altar can be on a tabletop, on the floor, or simply on your nightstand. It doesn't need to be fancy, because you can designate any space as sacred space. Amplify the love to your altar by adding things like flowers, crystals, religious items, books, or even little notes of love and intention. Place a white candle in the center of your altar. (If necessary, it can be battery-operated.)

Every day, sit for at least ten minutes and mentally repeat the day's prayer/mantra three times before going into silence. Sit in front of your altar with your eyes closed and your spine straight. Remain in silence, meditating on the mantra for as long as wish. My recommendation is to sit at least ten minutes.

Take a moment before getting up to stretch your body, slowly allowing the Divine energy to merge with yours. Journal your experience.

Day one prayer/mantra: "Angels of God, I invite you into my life."

Day two prayer/mantra: "Angels of God, I invite you to lift my energy."

Day three prayer/mantra: "Angels of God, guide me through this day."

Day four prayer/mantra: "Angels of God, assist me with [add your petition]."

Day five prayer/mantra: "Angels of God, fill my heart with Divine love and light."

Day six prayer/mantra: "Angels of God, illuminate the path for my highest and best good."

Day seven prayer/mantra: "Dearest Angels of God, thank you for your love and guidance throughout this week. I offer you my love and gratitude."

Journal Prompts:

After completing the exercise, use the following prompts to write about your experience in your journal.

- What prayer/mantra did you use today?
- What did you experience while using it?

There Are No Angels Outside of God

God is the giver of life, eternal love, the Father almighty. God makes up all of Heaven and Earth, what is seen and not seen. Everything exists in God, with God, and through God. Praying and honoring God is our birthright and an element of our free will. We remember God in the womb and as we are birthed into life.

As you do the exercises presented in this chapter, the pathway will open for you to continue to work with the Angels.

By simply setting sacred space within your being and in your life, you invite Divine guidance in, moment by moment. When we are able to shift our thoughts from being victims who have no control over a situation to truly loving ourselves and claiming our responsibility, we can separate ourselves from the energy of fear. When we choose to hold sacred space within our heart for someone who is hurting us, we shift our pattern of automatically receiving fear to learning to accept love instead. We also find ourselves able to honor the person as a teacher for our growth and see them with compassion, thus allowing the relationship to continue, or sometimes end, in the highest vibration of love.

Since the Angels are messengers of God, when we let them into our lives, we let God in too. This is transformational. You will quickly see how this shift in perspective changes everything.

CHAPTER TWO

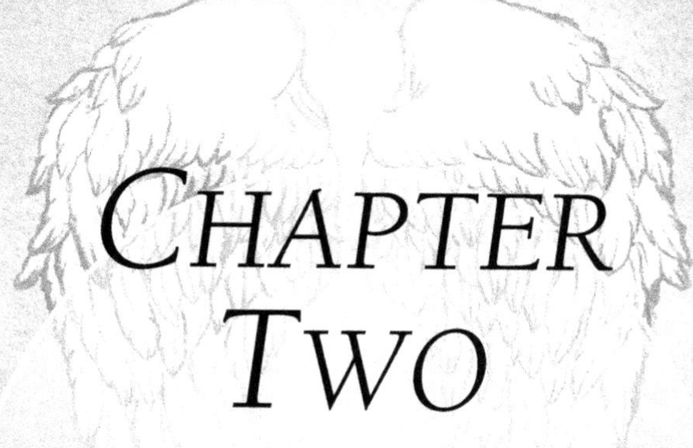

CHAPTER TWO

Knowing Our Soul's Truth

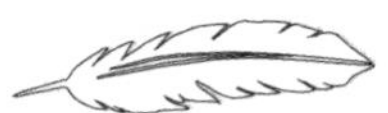

"You cannot believe in God until you believe in yourself."

— *SWAMI VIVEKANANDA*

Feeling Lost

I think it's safe to say that most of us get lost within our lives. I've witnessed colleagues, clients, family, and friends experience not knowing their true path in life, and I spent many years like this myself. It is a painful feeling to be lost, disconnected from our soul's truth. When this was my experience I was happy to some extent, but I was still lost. I had given my power away. Fear had me believing that I was undeserving and unworthy, that I wasn't smart because I hadn't done well in school or attended college. I felt unlovable. With such little self-respect, I unknowingly taught others to treat me the same way I was treating myself: like crap. I had to relearn how to love myself and, by doing so, I was able to take my power back—with pure Goddess style!

There are still moments when those old fear-based beliefs will creep back in, and I feel unworthy. Because I am an empath, my sense of knowing is like an open faucet that fills my body with the feelings and emotions of others. I can get caught up in what others think about me and almost immediately fall out of my Goddess alignment. These are times when I remind myself that the energy of others is not my truth. When I stay in connection with a client and the flow of their reading, their energy can convert into confusing feelings, sensations, and emotions within my body and mind. This is true for any one of us who is sensitive to the energy of others.

When Shmego and his fears jump in and claim those feelings, sensations and emotions as thoughts, he works to fill my mind with his endless, fearful lies. These lies connect the felt experience of another person to my own history, which in turn brings the feelings of unworthiness I just mentioned.

Exercise

I learned the following trick from the Angels. It helps me release the fear and surrender to love with faith. While keeping my connection to my client, I shut off the connection with Shmego, returning to my truth and Soul Self. I invite you to try it. It's a nifty trick that I use to turn off the negative aspects that accompany being an empath and stop fear in its tracks. You can do the following exercise wherever and whenever you need it!

Surrendering to Love:

Begin by setting your intention to surrender to God in the moment.

Close your eyes as you place the palms of your hands on your upper chest.

Breathe in through your nose until you feel your chest rise under your palms. Repeat this mantra: "I am the grace of God."

Hold the breath for a count of five before slowly releasing it out through your mouth. Repeat the mantra again: "I am the grace of God."

I recommend that you repeat this exercise three times in a row.

Journal Prompts:

After completing the exercise, use the following prompts to write about your experience in your journal.

- What intention did you set at the beginning of the exercise?
- What did you experience during the exercise?
- How did the exercise support you during your day?

Knowing Our Life Path

Owning who we are in this life comes easily for some people yet remains perplexing to others. Some know early on what they will do in their life; they seemingly just *know* their life's path. The rest of us aren't so sure, which puts us at risk for inadvertently giving our personal power away. This reduction of personal power happens little bits at a time as our feelings of unworthiness, self-loathing, or discomfort begin to change the way we view the world around us.

The people we know throughout our lives and the experiences we live through eventually become how we live and think. Our thoughts and actions are either healthy and love-based or they are laced with fear. Many spiritual teachers teach and talk about the fact that our thoughts turn into our reality. This is both a truth and a healing that the Angels say is vital for our happiness. I know that I've certainly fallen into judgment or victimhood when I've been pushed the wrong way! Most of us find that our judgment arises when we feel threatened or angry. Our relationships with others, and particularly the patterns within them, can also show us the truth about our own self-limiting beliefs and judgmental tones. This is because relationships are reflections.

Doing the "you work" to be the love for yourself first will ultimately guide you to see where love has always been available to you throughout your life. No matter how painful the event, with enough "you work" you will find the love rather than the pain you've chosen to see in its place. Since changing my point of view to focus on love and owning my personal power, I've been called an optimist by some—and it wasn't necessarily coming as a compliment. The way I see it, haters are gonna hate, and we don't have to take on their yucky energy!

Seeing the Negative and Being Brave

It is often easier for us to see the negative instead of the positive in any given situation. This is why it is so easy to judge ourselves and each other. I share the same exercise with my clients that the Angels guided me to do years ago when I began doing my "you work": make a list of "fear thoughts" versus "love thoughts."

I've witnessed the beneficial results this exercise has on an individual's life just by listing out their fear and love thoughts for one week. When doing this exercise, most people discover very quickly that they are fear addicts. When we change our thoughts from fear to love, our perception changes too. Then we can go back through our old stories and life events and witness where love was available to us instead of reliving that event from the standpoint of victimhood. By doing so, we heal the pain of the past.

I know this from my own experience. I became a mother at a young age; I was just twenty when I had my first baby and twenty-two when I had my second. Looking back, I see now that I was not present in my body most of those twenty-two years! I would fly out of my body or retreat within it to hide from the energy I was experiencing, a trait that is common among both empaths and sensitive souls. But I knew one thing for sure: I wanted to be a mother.

My first baby was delivered via an emergency Cesarean section and left me with more than one scar—one physical, and the other emotional, as I'd almost lost my baby during labor. I was therefore quite fearful the second time around. As it turned out, I had a completely different delivery. In the middle of a contraction, the doctor saw that I was disconnected from my body. He brought out a mirror so I could connect with what was happening, not only with my body but also with the labor itself. The problem was that I had been going through the motions of pushing yet was having little success. The pain was really intense, and I wasn't making much progress. It was too late for any pain medication, and I was actually feeling like giving up because in my mind, my pelvic bone was either going to burn apart or break in half. The doctor brought out the mirror and told me he wanted me to watch the next contraction before I pushed. I was horrified. Was he serious? He really wanted me to look down there—at that pain? *I can't look at that pain,* I thought. I had to hold it in; that's what I'd always done. *He's crazy, and I will not follow along with crazy.*

I know now that his point was to have me be present not only in the moment but also in my body. He knew that this would help me be more effective in my laboring; he was, in essence, being the love I needed at that moment. But I was horrified, and my decision was to stay hidden within and to not look pain in the eye. Lo and behold, I finally made it through the delivery without looking in that horrid, stupid mirror, and gave birth to a beautiful baby boy.

I was clearly not ready to be awakened. More than thirty years later, I once again find myself called to look into that proverbial mirror. This time the mirror is the reflection of my truth and why I keep hiding the true source of who I am now that fear has been stripped away. I hide behind shy, introverted behaviors to avoid speaking my truth to family and friends who know that old version of me. I cannot tell you how many of these close old pals I've known through the years, some of whom are in my family, say, "Jeanne, how come I didn't know you are a medium?" The truth is that I have been worried that they would judge me and, in that judgment, choose not to love me. Schmego's twisted fear-based illusion had me believe that they would leave me, taking their love and running far, far away. Yet now I see the mirror of truth reflecting back at me, telling me that my fear is a judgment of others. So now in this mirror of truth, of love, of being whole, I find that I have to be both vulnerable and brave enough to share my story. I have to look right at the pain that accompanies my fear of not being loved; I have to push through it anyway.

I was pondering all these illusions when the Angels illuminated my soul path. I was sitting at the edge of the gynecologist's table, wearing a paper robe. I stared at the stirrups at the end of the table, my dangling legs jittering nervously as I awaited the doctor's arrival. I knew I had to lie back and put my feet in the stirrups. And, just like when I was delivering my babies, I sensed a birthing happening. I was suddenly flooded with the feelings of just how uncomfortable it was to be there on that table. I thought, *Here you are again, Jeanne. You've got to put your feet in those darn stirrups, with only this thin paper robe to clench to for protection. Now this is vulnerability: in seconds you'll be heels high in this awkward moment.*

It was there, in all my uneasiness, when I was feeling stripped down and exposed, that I became acutely aware I was actually experiencing the energy of bravery. Yes, I was vulnerable, but I paired that vulnerability with my bravery to stand in my truth—or, in this case, lie with my feet in those stupid stirrups. I realized that moments like those are when the layers of the ego-self are peeled away.

Being exposed is something I've generally tried to avoid, often by running away. Maybe you've experienced running away as well. But now I am choosing love and staying in the moment rather than retreating. Faith is what supports and holds me in that love, and that's exactly what I wish for you as well. You don't have to be at the gynecologist's office to find your bravery, but it just so happened to be the place where mine showed up. Go figure.

Grief, Trauma and Vulnerability

None of us really wants to feel exposed. Yet when we stay in our vulnerability long enough, we actually start to feel safe because we realize it isn't the situation that protects us: it's our own inner power. It is here in this uncertain and lonely moment of being exposed and uncomfortable that the authenticity of who we are can begin to shine brightly. Love embraces all of our brokenness. With faithful steadiness and security, it supports us to withstand any fearful moment.

To get to this point, we must be willing to change how we see our pain. We have to be ready to spend the time needed to gaze in the mirror and give value to whatever our reflection is waiting to teach us. It is here that our greatness will rise to the surface, out of the ashes of our pain.

I have a term for this process when we look at our life with a new gaze:

owl vision. Owl eyes will give us a 360-degree view of our past pains. Using this method to become a witness or spectator of our suffering is a beautiful way of validating our feelings. It can help us notice where love was available and what lesson can be taken away from the situation.

Traumas, like grief, don't just go away. There is a new normal that welcomes itself into our life once we've changed the position in which we are standing. It boils down to this: either we are a victim who comes from the standpoint of "I am grief" or we are an empowered being who is experiencing grief and who understands, "I have grief."

Grief, as the Angels have shown me, can best be categorized into what I call the "Four Es."

1. ***Emotional.*** This is how we feel grief within our body. Emotions are energetic tones stored in our being, similar to how muscles have memory and can return to shape. The Angels say our emotions are imprinted the same way. Our senses are the trigger recalling our emotional memory to come to the surface.

2. ***Energetic.*** We can witness the energy tones of grief through the highs and lows we experience through feeling the emotional waves of our grief.

3. ***Experience.*** We all experience grief on our own personal level. Our connection to a particular grief can stay with us for as long as it takes for our healing to come forward.

4. ***Exhaustion.*** This is how our bodies respond to the energy, emotions, and experience of grief.

The confusing part is that the Four Es of grief are intertwined and can be felt simultaneously. In any case, knowing the separate factors at play helps us to be aware of the signs and know when to get ourselves help.

Exercise

This exercise can help change how to see your reflection.

360-Degree Reflection:

Find a peaceful spot to meditate with your journal and pen by your side.

Say the following prayer: "Dear God, I ask that you surround and embrace me in Your Divine holy love and that Your loving light deflects all fear away from my gaze. Let me use my owl vision to see myself as pure love."

Begin cycle breathing as you adjust your body into a comfortable position, keeping your spine straight. Close your eyes and relax your tongue away from the roof of your mouth.

Let your thoughts float by as you engage your inner vision and bring your awareness to your third eye chakra.

Relax your body with each breath as you notice that your third eye opens to the light of God shining inward.

Allow your eyes to shift behind your eyelids. As you adjust your focus back to your third eye, notice the range in which you are looking outward has increased.

Now gently shift your eyes down toward your chin, then to the back of your head, finally resting upward at the crown of your head. This awakens the connection to your crown chakra, where Divine love flows into your third eye. Bring your vision outward and around you, as if you were in a 360-degree movie theater.

Playing on the movie screen is the memory of a time when you were hurt. Not only can you see yourself: you can see all the people who were around you, as well as their feelings and emotions.

It is in this place that you call on God to shine the light of love that reflects the truth, the lessons, and clarity you need to heal.

Stay in this moment for as long as you need. Be still.

Do not worry if you only saw small snippets or even became afraid and left the meditation early. Healing takes time. Take all the time you need and revisit this meditation when you are ready.

When you have absorbed all that you can at this time, gently move your body and begin to write your experience down in your journal.

Journal:

Write in your journal about how you are feeling and any experiences you had.

Grief's Timeline

A person can only love as the measure in which they love themselves. We must love ourselves ***Holy***. Only then will our relationship with self and others grow.

Knowing our soul's truth comes from aligning with our Soul Self while doing our "you work" to heal the suffering that has gathered over time from our life experiences. Our past is carried within our body, creating feelings and emotions that separate us from love. Shame, sorrow, and self-pity are the constraints that hold our pain and grief in place. Our outer world reflects the energetic state of our inner being. The good news is that when healed, our being releases that energy, and without these feelings we are free to experience a new way of living. This is the miracle that comes when we bravely take the time to do the "you work", to self-love and heal. And I think it's very important for all of us to know and really comprehend that there is no right or wrong time to heal, because there are no time restraints in Heaven, and the Angels show that the same applies for healing our grief. Healing happens when we can actively engage in addressing grief within our own time frame.

CHAPTER THREE

CHAPTER THREE

Divine Christ Energy

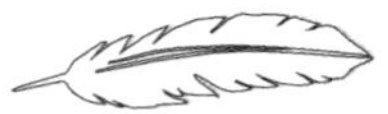

"Long ago, at many times and in many ways, God spoke to our fathers by the prophets, but in these last days he has spoken to us by his Son, whom he appointed the heir of all things, through whom also he created the world. He is the radiance of the glory of God and the exact imprint of his nature, and he upholds the universe by the word of his power. After making purification for sins, he sat down at the right hand of the Majesty on high, having become as much superior to angels as the name he has inherited is more excellent than theirs."

— *HEBREWS 1:1–4 ESV*

It's time to shed some light on our beautiful path in this life. A channeled message I received from God says, "Pray unto Me, through My Son, the Holy Spirit, Angels and archangels, and I will answer so you may find peace, comfort, and guidance. Pray unto Me for your weaknesses and I will make you whole. Pray unto Me your sins and you shall be set free. In all things see Me, and in all things I see you. Blessed be all who rejoice in the Glory of God."

Pray for what you think you need and you will be left feeling empty; pray for God's will for you and all of your needs will be met. There are no perfect prayers or a right way of talking to God. He is always available to listen and hear our heart's desires, questions, and petitions at any given moment.

God and His almighty communion of holy spiritual beings are how I first began to open the door to work with the Angels. You may notice your inner connection to the Divine through religion or outside of it. The starting point of our soul's truth and knowing comes with clearing up our life from fear's energy that causes us to become beings who are stuck and isolated. As I began clearing up my fearful thoughts and ways, I was able to welcome back in my connection to the Holy Spirit.

The holy trinity is representative of the power of the holy three: the Father, the Son, and the Holy Spirit, the three energies that are God. Then, of course, there is the mystical and Divine nature of the number three and Jesus's energy. Jesus lived thirty-three years; He prayed three times before His arrest; His crucifixion began on the third hour of the day and ended on the ninth hour; and He rose from the dead on the third day.

It is through prayer that we can speak to God, Jesus, and other holy beings about our worries, cares and concerns for self and for others. It is through meditation and journaling that the Divine answers us. In my meditation, Jesus taught me the three holy Christ points. The hands are the first point, the feet are the second, and the heart and lung area are the third. The three Christ points are connection points or, as some call them, chakra points. Healers who work with God's energy have open Christ points. These are the points at which the healer connects to the mystical, Divine, and miraculous energy of God, Jesus, and the Holy Spirit. The three Christ points are not taught to us by someone else; they are gifts that are bestowed onto the soul. We will awaken to owning our place in this life and walking our rightful path when we open and meditate on our Christ points.

The number three has significant meaning in other religions and spiritual studies as well. It's often considered a lucky number. There are popular sayings we often use, such as "The third time's the charm" or "Three strikes and you're out." We can also connect to a deeper meaning with the number three when we reference it to our personal life such as the past, present, and future; the mind, body, and soul; or even birth, life, and death. There are also many who believe and say that things always happen in threes.

Fear and Healing

Some souls are born as healers. Their journey in this life is to shine their light outward and connect their Christ points to the path of healing. Many of them will often deny this energy out of fear and shame, which is the work of evil against the holy truth. This keeps the healer hidden by self-doubt, worry, denial, and judgment, which can lead them to closing the connection to the Divine energy. Evil will work hard to maintain a detachment from God, religion, or Source and will wield its power to keep the healer from standing in their rightful path.

Fear can also become the starting point for addictions to take hold. Many healers are led to a deeper hiding place where self-loathing actions, such as addictions, are the pathways for numbing what we don't fully understand about our unique gift. This can end up leading to a separation from our Soul Self. Healers, empaths, and sensitive souls are here to share the love of God with others. But many instead end up consumed by grief, guilt, shame, blame, and all that fear does to make them hide or play small. That way, they aren't able to shine or share Divine love.

My client-turned-friend Norma is an example of a healer who was plagued by fear and did not understand her calling as a healer. The first time I channeled Jesus without reservation or fear was during a session with Norma.

Norma had been coming for healing sessions regularly over the span of two years. She was struggling with her abilities as an empath and was receiving relentless confusing energy. She was also dealing with the aftermath of a painful divorce and suffering PTSD from her personal experience with the Sandy Hook shootings. Norma's daughter had been in the afternoon kindergarten class at Sandy Hook Elementary. Fortunately, she was not in attendance during the time the shootings took place, but the experience still altered their lives profoundly because it was just so close to home.

Not only did Norma not know how to heal the endless guilt and despair she felt, she was also unable to shut off the energy she was constantly feeling, or "downloading," as she put it. Her fears were magnified by the energy she picked up in her field of work as a psychiatric nurse. Norma entered my healing room with a dark energy lurking around her. As we began the session I called on the Angels, asking for God's love and protection to surround us both. I typically begin my healing sessions at the feet. This allows me to immediately connect with my client's energy and see their vibrational state. Upon grasping Norma's feet, I was shown the lull in her energy as my body swayed to the left. This is how I am shown that a person is stuck in a logical, overthinking mind. I also felt a depletion that spoke of suicidal thoughts. As my body swayed in her energy, the air shifted in the room. I called on Jesus to help me.

In an instant I began speaking, but not of my own accord; the words were not mine. I heard myself saying words of love, compassion, and truth about how Norma was worthy beyond her limited self-belief and how this limiting belief only acted as a shield to block love. I recognized that Jesus was speaking through me. Jesus spoke of matters beyond the current moment and how Norma could open her thought system in a new and different energetic way in order to revitalize her soul's essence. The room was transformed before my earthly eyes to a heavenly healing sanctuary. Illuminated celestial beings glided effortlessly in a rhythmic harmonious pattern as time stood still. The angelic beings began placing what appeared to be rays of color shaped in unfamiliar symbols into Norma's heart center. As the session progressed, I felt my being and the room return to normal. I looked at Norma as she spoke: "Did you hear Jesus speaking through you?" She, too, had recognized the voice as that of Jesus. I felt that I was both a witness and a participant in what had just taken place. Neither of us had ever experienced such a holy moment.

After receiving a profound healing from this divinely channeled message,

Norma was able to move out of the stagnant way of living that had consumed her in the wake of the shooting—but only for a short time. It came through to me from a shamanic healer that Norma was seeking answers and guidance from other sources as well. The Angels showed me that Norma was not yet ready to merge with the profound changes that were needed to align with her Soul Self path; fear was burdening her day and night. We texted several times before she came to see me for another healing session, again desperate to relieve the intense energy she was witnessing both within her body and visually. Upon seeing her again, I was immediately concerned; I felt she was in danger of losing her sense of self. I turned my concerns over to Jesus, asking for assistance so I could be a clear vessel for truth and guidance for Norma.

As she lay on the table with tears streaming down her face, talking of extraterrestrial beings and lights that kept her awake and nagged at her for days at a time, the compassion and love from inside my being burst from my heart to hers. Led by the Divine, I calmly laid my hands upon her feet to connect and slowly moved to the crown of her head. I pleaded with Jesus to help her. And then, just like before, I felt Jesus in the room, this time not talking through me, rather talking to me as He stood next to Norma and ever so gently gestured to her head. Jesus said she had a mass, a tumor causing the lights and bursts of unsteady energy. He said a CT scan was needed, but surgery or radiation were not. As he slowly faded into the veil and the room returned to its natural state, I gently shared with Norma the messages I had received. She, too, had felt Jesus' presence. I described what I'd seen about the nature of the mass and explained that the Angels had assured me it could be healed with medicinal mushrooms and a shift in diet. Norma left and went directly to the hospital for a CT scan. The ER doctor confirmed the Divine message: Norma had a tumor called a *jugular foramen schwannoma* and a pineal gland cyst.

Of course, the medical world is not always tuned in to Divine healing, and it's certainly not commonly understood yet that each person can heal their own mind, body, and soul. Norma still struggles between fear, the earthly world of chaos and the need for knowledge, and her innate trust in love and Divine truth. She gets annual brain scans to watch for new growth or changes in the tumor. Her healing journey has not been an easy one. But she continues on, raising her daughter, as a single mom, and working full time. The tumor remains stable. Her daughter is now a beautiful, happy preteen. And my friend Norma is a beautiful soul whose shining light glows brightly beyond the material world! Norma recently shared her healing story with the audience of my *Angels Don't Lie* show. You can listen to it at jeannestreet.com/jesus-speaks/.

Healing requires full faith, but this faith is not easily utilized when fear has a hold over one's thoughts. The power we have over fear is exercised by our decision to choose love. By aligning with the Divine and connecting to love and compassion moment by moment, our thoughts will shift from fear to love. Learning to recognize fear and live in our soul alignment are achievable by following the twelve Goddess principles. Living in soul alignment is a course of action that we can choose in each moment. It helps us release fear's grip and allow truth, love, and light to become our everyday joy.

Christ Points and Chakras

I spoke of the Christ points earlier. These are a known phenomenon. Most people have experienced a warm surge of energy in the palms of their hands at some point. This is the best way that I can describe the sensation of having the Christ points open and flowing with Divine energy. Our palms and the soles of our feet often start to tingle slightly, and then we feel warm vibrating energy flowing outward. Though what I am describing is not about religion, there is a simplistic truth that we should address, and that is our belief and relationship with God and Jesus. As we know, Jesus is the Son of God. He spent his life teaching, guiding, and helping those in need, and he also performed miraculous healings. If we are able to accept these Divine truths and surrender our will to God's love, we can connect to His healing energy. Working with our Christ points is similar to working with our chakra energy centers. We open these centers by inviting the Divine in through prayer, intent, and angelic guidance. Then the energy will open, balance, and flow through us.

The points in the feet connect us to our life and time in the physical world. The Soul Self is an infinite energy source that can connect through the veil. As humans, we are both here in the physical world and in the spiritual world through our soul connection. Most people are separate from their Soul Self. They move through life unaware of their soul's purpose, confused and undirected. This separation occurs for various reasons within our soul's life.

We can connect to our Soul Self by starting with the Christ points located in the soles of our feet. Doing so allows us to stand confidently in any moment. By opening our Christ points, we are agreeing to connect with our Goddess truths with faith, confidence, and self-love. There is nothing more beautiful and profound than seeing another standing in alignment with their Soul Self.

Let me break it down a bit further.

There are seven main chakra points in the body. The first, the root chakra, is located between our hips at the base of our spine. The root chakra governs our lower organs, including our lower extremities, and is associated with the beginning of life. When we have experienced childhood trauma or the early onset of anger, we will be disconnected from our true feelings, and this will show up in the root chakra. When opened and balanced, this chakra will transform our pain from fear to love and lead us to forgiveness and compassion. When we take this a step further and open the Christ point in the soles of our feet, we then can heal the pains and burdens on a deeper level. Opening our Christ points illuminates what no longer serves us, as we are fully supported by standing firmly with God, knowing our soul's value and claiming our place here on Earth.

There is one main fact that I want you to always remember: you are meant to be here! Aligning our mind, body, and soul so we can work with Jesus and this mystical, Divine healing energy can absolutely transform our lives in miraculous ways. To help with this, I offer you the following exercise to help open your root chakra and the Christ points in your feet.

Exercise

This meditation and journal exercise will help you connect with your lower root chakra.

Connecting to Your Root Chakra:

Remove your shoes so your feet are bare. Then say the following prayer of intention: "Dear God, shower me with Your Divine light and love as I connect my body, mind, and soul with you. I ask for angelic assistance to connect my chakra points to Divine love."

Close your eyes and plant your feet firmly on the ground as you slowly inhale and exhale deeply several times.

Allow your body to relax and let go of any tension in your neck, shoulders, and arms as you inhale. Then as you exhale, slowly bring your attention first to your crown then to your third eye chakra. With your intent and awareness, invite these chakras to open and merge with Divine energy.

Notice how your breath merges with Divine energy as you inhale and exhale. Then with an inhale, feel your lungs and belly fill completely, opening your throat and heart chakra points. Exhale completely.

With your next inhale, bring your breath to your abdomen, allowing the breath to move into your solar plexus and sacral chakra.

As you continue breathing even deeper, let your breath descend into your hip area, connecting to your root chakra.

Now bring your awareness to your legs and allow the energy to move past any blocks that may be there. Notice your feet as you inhale, bringing your breath all the way down to the soles. Feel your feet connect to your breath. Feel the sensations of the Divine energy expanding in your body. "Nancy Drew it!" Become a detective of how, what, and why your senses are being activated. This will help you distinguish how Spirit is guiding you.

Sit here with your feet connected to your place on Earth and be still as long as you need.

Journal Prompts:

After completing the exercise, use the following prompts to write about your experience in your journal.

- Describe the Divine energy you feel.
- Describe any sensations associated with each of your chakra points.
- What did you notice when you brought your breath to your root chakra?
- How do you feel now?

Return to this meditation anytime you feel disconnected from your light.

The Role of Faith

Faith is the pathway to restoring the separation from the source of who we are to our authentic Soul Self. Faith restores the imbalance of fearful energy to the rightful loving Divine truth. It's a great way to turn off Shmego's constant fear tactics!

Janie's story illustrates the role faith plays in healing. She came for a reading one cold February day. I met her by the stairway when she arrived for her session. I was immediately overcome with the heaviness of her grief. The Angels showed me that Janie was in a delicate state by impressing an eggshell in my mind. I immediately knew that this was a sign to move slowly and keep my voice low.

I escorted Janie into my office where I offered her tea or water. "Water," she said in a curt, low tone. I excused myself to go and get a freshwater bottle. During my absence, the Angels again impressed the importance of being gentle and even toned with Janie. I returned to the office and I could feel her anxiety and pain. The energy surrounding her was a motionless, muddy-colored wave.

I began the session, as I always do, with an explanation of how I do my readings and how I sometimes use my journal to write down the impressions Spirit is sending me. I also interpret the signs, symbols, feelings, and emotions within my body as I relay and connect the messages to my clients. I let

Janie know that she could ask questions at any time. I began to scribe the first impressions Spirit offered. The word "mother" came through, along with a feeling of desperation. I relayed this message and in a snappy voice, Janie replied, "My mother is not dead." As I continued, Spirit kept repeating the message "mother" in the same tone. I told this to Janie, explaining that it was perhaps something about her relationship with her mom. Janie cut me off by saying, "I am not here to talk about my mother." I could feel the tension rising and Janie's body stiffen. I pleaded with Spirit to throw me a bone with something more so I could help this poor grieving woman, who was obviously in a great deal of pain. But Spirit only repeated "mother." So once again I explained that I was being guided to ask or talk about the idea of mothers—either her as a mother, or her own mother. Janie shook her head, again saying, "That is not why I came here," this time with tears in her eyes.

I spoke calmly as Spirit moved through me to explain that the impressions I get are the pathway inviting the Divine flow to open, and that when we are blocking the energy with fear or grief, we can miss the message's meaning. I told Janie that although I had never experienced this type of reading where I was unable to deliver what Spirit was guiding me to give to my client, I would not charge her or waste her time if she was not happy. As I spoke these words, I was even more confident in the message Spirit was giving me. I knew that this session was too painful and too soon after a great loss for Janie to sit through. She looked up at me with eyes of sorrow, eyes that spoke of pain and despair as she reached for her purse and repeated the words, "You won't charge me?" I repeated that I would not, speaking with assurance that I trust what I am shown and if it wasn't meant to be me, Spirit would bring forward another soul to deliver the message to Janie.

Janie quickly picked up her belongings and headed for the stairs. I wished her well. As she left the studio without looking back, I could hear her sobbing. My heart ached for her. I returned to my office to sit in a prayer meditation and asked the Angels to surround Janie with love and gentle guidance.

Two weeks later, I received a phone call. I did not recognize her voice at first; she sounded like a completely different person. Janie explained, "I just had to call you to tell you that I know what you were trying to tell me now. I had lost my son and wanted to only hear from him that day. Later, when I got home from your studio, the mother of his fiancé phoned me. She told me that her daughter had just passed away. I was not ready to hear the words you were speaking. I had no idea at the time that it was my son and future daughter-in-law trying to talk to me."

Janie told me she had booked a reading with another medium just after seeing me. This medium delivered the same message, but this time she was open to receive. Janie wanted to apologize for how she left that day. She was so distraught over her son's passing she was not able to hear that he was coming through, calling to her from Heaven: "Mother!"

I was happy to be able to extend my gratitude to Janie and to explain that I have learned to always trust the messages I get, and that I know what I know simply because Angels don't lie.

Janie returned a year later for a reading. This time she was fully open to hearing and receiving the loving messages that awaited her.

"The lowly he sets on high, and those who mourn are lifted to safety."

—JOB 5:11 NIV

The Archangels

Now, my friend, I will share with you my personal connection with the archangels and how they have revealed themselves to me. At the end of this section, I will guide you through a connection meditation so you can better get to know the archangels and begin your own personal relationship with them.

Keep in mind that Shmego will do his job of inducing fear and limiting thoughts where we have the slightest of doubts. To combat Shmego's relentless fear tones, we must stay connected with God in love and faith. Try saying the following prayer before reading this section and see if you notice Shmego sneaking in.

> **Prayer of Protection:** *"Dear God, please surround me with Your white light of love and protection, protecting me from fear's limiting energy, and gently guide me throughout the following passages so that I may experience Your glory through knowing the archangels. Amen."*

Archangels, I have come to know, are dutiful when called upon and emit the purest Godlike energy. Just as there is a hierarchy of celestial beings to call upon, there are specific reasons that justify assistance from the archangels. There is free will to remember, of course, and there is always the will of God to keep in mind. As the Lord's Prayer goes, "Thy will be done." Similar to all Angels, archangels can appear as a communion of energy, not necessarily as a singular being. Archangels are seated closest to God. They are vastly expansive, beyond human mathematical equations, and contain an infinite number of "beings" that make up their celestial energy.

Archangels can appear one at a time or as a communion of the same tone and energy, which is why they will appear larger than life. The archangels I share with you here are a few of whom I have connected with personally. The four I have chosen to share with you are not the only archangels I work with. I chose these four because of my heritage and connection with Christianity. Many religions speak of archangels and their work, and as there are multitudes of different religions, there are also numerous teachings about the many different archangels.

Archangel Michael. In Hebrew, Michael's name means "the one who is like God." Michael takes form as a warrior ready to battle the forces of the darkness. His form is large, strong and powerful. His energy is friendly, kind, forgiving, and relentless in the pursuit of protection and honor. He will shoulder your pain to help lift you out of the trenches of life's misery. Archangel Michael will protect you with the sword of God's love while shielding you from the darkness, allowing Divine light to touch you.

When we are in need of protection for ourselves or a loved one, we need only close our eyes, pray to God, and invite Archangel Michael into our lives through a prayer, asking for what we need in our prayer petition with pure intention and love.

> **For example:** *"Dear God, please send Archangel Michael to my side, as I am in need of protection and love to guide me through writing this book. Please surround me with your white light of unending love and protect me from fear and its illusions. Amen."*

When I call on Archangel Michael, I feel his energy as a large man—larger than life, similar to what I imagine a celestial linebacker would be—who is tall and unwavering. Archangel Michael's energy is blue in color and feels kind and soft, like a true friend you have known for your whole life and who would protect you from any bully. Yet Archangel Michael is also a no-nonsense being and will call us out if we have moved off our soul's path. Amethyst crystals are known to help with connecting to Archangel Michael.

Archangel Gabriel. In Hebrew, Gabriel means "God is my strength." This archangel takes form as a loyal messenger, eager to deliver truth with kindness, gentleness, and ease. Archangel Gabriel delivers messages only in accordance with God's will. Archangel Gabriel's loyal yellow tone and loving nature will empower our ability to speak truth from the heart center, also known as the seat of our soul.

When we are in need of receiving or delivering truth or a message, we can call upon Archangel Gabriel to aid us in softening our tone and aligning with our soul's truth to receive or deliver our message with Divine love.

> **For example:** *"Dear God, please send Archangel Gabriel to help me deliver the Divine truth and messages meant for the highest and best good of all who find their way to this book. Let Your will be done with the guidance of Archangel Gabriel. Amen."*

When I call on Archangel Gabriel, he appears large with both female and male energy in balance, like the yin and yang of a human. Archangel

Gabriel's energy is soft yet electrifying, exuding Divine love and truth. Archangel Gabriel will softly deliver even the hardest message we can imagine, and it will be delivered and received with Divine holy love. Try using a citrine crystal to aid in the connection to Archangel Gabriel.

Archangel Raphael. In Hebrew, Raphael means "God heals." This archangel takes the form of trusted intellect. He exudes knowledge of many subjects and matters dealing with the well-being of the human condition. Tried-and-true Archangel Raphael will bear witness to our pain and suffering to better guide us toward love's light and healing.

When we are in need of healing, we can call on Archangel Raphael to assist us on our journey to well-being.

> ***For example:*** *"Dear God, please send Archangel Raphael to assist me in balancing my physical, mental, and spiritual energy while writing. Help me to be in my highest vibrational energy and well-being as I channel all these loving messages. Amen."*

When I call on Archangel Raphael, he appears like a tall, strong, all-knowing professor of medicine filled with green energy. Archangel Raphael's energy realigns the false with the Divine truth, and his reassurance of love will gently support our healing journey. Emerald or green crystals will aid our connection to Archangel Raphael.

Archangel Uriel. In Hebrew, Uriel means "God is my light." This archangel takes the form wisdom would if wisdom were a man. Archangel Uriel's bright vibrant energy forms a shield of reddish light around him. Archangel Uriel carries with him the wisdom, knowledge, and kindness of God's will. Archangel Uriel will help you sort out your fearful lower energy thought system and help you to realign with God's truth. Justice will prevail with Archangel Uriel by your side. Amber is the crystal associated with connecting to Archangel Uriel.

When we are in need of a higher wisdom or justice, we can call on Archangel Uriel to swiftly guide us with the all-knowing truth of God's will.

For example: *"Dear God, I ask that you please send Your loyal guardian of wisdom and knowledge, Archangel Uriel, to assist me as I write about Your kingdom. May I be the vessel and voice to deliver Your Divine and holy messages. Amen."*

When I call on Archangel Uriel, he appears strong and sturdy, like royalty. His armor is God's light, which glistens from his eyes. Archangel Uriel's wisdom exudes from his holy presence. I am immediately comforted by the redirection of the loving wisdom he offers.

The following is just one of the connection meditations you can use to connect with the archangels. For more meditations, visit **believeangels.com**.

Exercise

To begin, choose which archangel you will work with in your mediation. You will work with one chakra at a time, and slowly reflect on each of your senses before moving to the next chakra. "Nancy Drew it!"

As a reminder, the seven chakras are:

- The root chakra, located at the base of your spine.
- The sacral chakra, located below the belly button.
- The solar plexus chakra, located below your rib cage.
- The heart chakra, located in the center of your chest.
- The throat chakra, located in the center of your neck.
- The third eye chakra, located between your eyebrows.
- The crown chakra, located at the top of your head.

Inviting the Archangel into your Chakras:

Begin by setting your intention to surrender to God in the moment.

Close your eyes as you place the palms of your hands on your upper chest.

Say a prayer of love and gratitude as you begin calling in your archangel of choice. Then close your eyes and take a deep, slow breath in through your nose as you silently count to ten, holding the breath in, before slowly exhaling to the count of ten.

Breathe to this count several times as you relax your muscles and entire body. Allow your mind to just be.

Keep your focus on your breath and the count as you let go.

Bring your awareness to your root chakra.

In your mind's eye, visualize the energy within the chakra center and invite your archangel to align this chakra with Source. Continue for a few more breath cycles and then move to the sacral chakra. Continue like this all the way up to the crown chakra.

Journal Prompts:

After completing the exercise, use the following prompts to write about your experience in your journal.

- What did you see in each chakra point?
- What did your senses experience?
- Which archangel did you choose, and what was your experience with them?

When to Call the Archangels

Calling on the archangels for guidance or protection during our challenging times, or to assist a loved one in need, will enhance the power of our prayers and the love in our lives. These celestial beings of Divine love from God are at our fingertips at any given moment; we need only call on them and they will arrive.

There are simple ways to incorporate calling on the archangels and opening our Christ points, infusing them into our spiritual practice. First, it's important to understand that what we are talking about here is a form of energy healing for our highest and best good. By opening our Christ points in the palms of our hands and gently rubbing our palms together while calling on the archangels, we can channel Divine energy. We can also call on the archangels and Divine energy to send prayers to both ourselves and others. This practice can also help to relieve physical pain if we place our palms over the area of discomfort. We can also call on Divine energy for gently relieving anxiety or even to calm a fussy baby. There are endless situations where this source of love can be of use.

Healers, doctors, nurses, bodyworkers, therapists, and countless other types of practitioners can also utilize their Christ points to offer Divine energy healing to enhance their work. When these and other healing modalities are combined with opening the Christ points and the Divine energy flow, a magnificent shift in energy occurs for both the healer and the one being healed.

CHAPTER FOUR

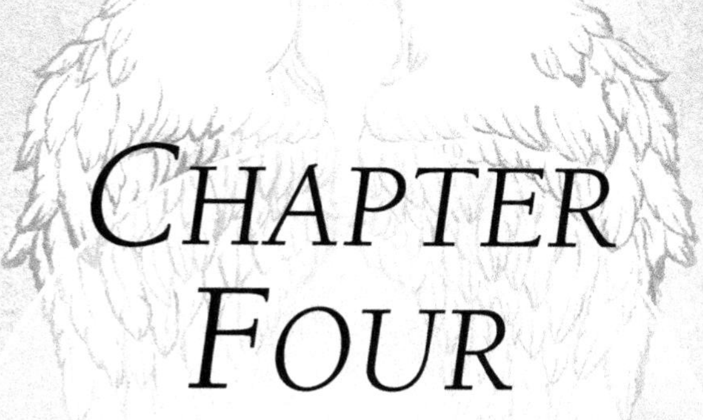

CHAPTER FOUR

Our Highest Good

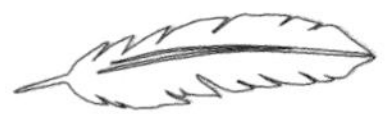

Our hearts reveal the core of who we are and what we stand for. The Divine knows this truth and is always guiding us to experience challenges that form the essence of our lives. Our character is what God is intent on building. Becoming our Soul Self isn't about losing ourselves or giving up; it's about becoming one with love, which is Source itself.

Angels are guiding us even when we are not aware of it. Gently, without force, they bring things to our awareness that will serve our highest good. Books, music, art, cooking, classes, people—the list of ways the Divine will gift us just the right energy to propel us forward in our alignment is endless. Sometimes, if and when we are so far out of alignment, the Angels have to pull out the "big dogs" for our highest and best good. They have to get our attention fast!

Here's another truth: Most people go through their day without once connecting to their Soul Self. This is an incredibly sad thing, because our Soul Self is freakin' awesome!

For instance, I was not seeing the signs that the Angels were sending my way to prompt me to talk about Father Al on my radio show. Father Al is the dearly departed friend who married my husband and me back in 1985. His wedding sermon was about real love, and he tied together our special day with a quote from the classic children's book *The Velveteen Rabbit* by Margery Williams: "Real isn't how you are made; it's a thing that happens to you." In 2011, although Father Al was retired and ninety-three years old, we were blessed to have him repeat this memorable sermon for our son and daughter-in-law's wedding.

Years later, after he had crossed over to Heaven, I started seeing images of Father Al in different places. At first I came across some old photos of him, and then I started seeing people who looked like him. One day, I noticed that my right thumbnail looked just as his did. Throughout my life, Spirit has often used hands as a sign to imprint the soul and the type of work that person does or did in this life. I was so busy working on my website and calendar of upcoming events that I did not slow down and take the time to connect with the message coming from Spirit and Father Al, who were so lovingly trying to guide me. What happened instead was that the Angels used a physical being, an earth messenger, to deliver the guidance instead.

I was texting with my friend Colleen when, out of the blue, she asked if I had a show topic yet for the next episode of the *Angels Don't Lie* radio show. I replied that I was still unsure but was thinking along the lines of higher perspective. The next text she wrote said, "But it feels real when we tap into Source and feel the love and see the perfection. It takes me back to the 'Believing Is Seeing' blog you wrote, which was so powerful for me. Maybe you can bring in the Velveteen Rabbit somehow!" Bingo! There it was, the connection to the message the Angels were trying to send me. I hadn't been listening, so they pulled out the "big dogs"! I finally understood why I had been seeing Father Al's face and hands and reminiscing on the fond memories of times spent with him. I intuitively knew what to do next: stop, drop and pray! I hit my yoga mat and allowed the message to guide me as I let go of control and fear that was stifling my connection to Spirit. I felt Divine love flowing through me, melting away the disconnect and restoring the Divine guidance.

Free Will, the Masculine and the Feminine

Angels cannot interfere with free will. One reason this is true is that you, I, and each living soul are all here to learn lessons, to grow and heal. Our souls have been given free will to choose. Choosing our path is our soul's destiny; we can align with truth or with fear. In any given moment we can choose to go it alone, follow fear or to choose love, and in doing so we choose God. God wants us to live with love, abundance, and joy. These are all readily available for us when we choose them.

When we put into perspective that our life lessons, pain, and suffering are the challenges our soul must go through in order to remember, grow, and remain connected to God and Divine love, we can better understand our purpose is to be the love our soul is seeking.

Our soul is here to be challenged, to learn valuable lessons, and to expand from these moments. Our soul's journey in this life is to grow with love and expand in consciousness. As we grow and learn to embrace love by connecting with God, our soul transforms energetically and comes into alignment. This means our souls are here in our body and are also connected with God. Remember earlier when we talked about our soul being infinite? This is how we connect our earthly self with our Soul Self, our Goddess Soul Self.

Let me clarify the illusion that the word "Goddess" refers only to women. This is a misconception. You see, everyone has both masculine and feminine energy within them. The Divine masculine side is the logical, analytical, and ego side. Ego is formed from our thoughts; it's the logical, matter-of-fact, emotionally responsive side of us. The Divine feminine side is the spiritual, compassionate, understanding, love-flowing side. When the two energies work together, Divine love comes into balance—but when one is more dominant than the other, chaos reigns.

> *"The heart of the wise inclines to the right, but the heart of the fool to the left."*
>
> — *ECCLESIASTES 10:2 NIV*

The Divine masculine, which is the logical left side of our body, is off-balance when it is controlled by fear. Our need for proof, knowledge, and righteousness arises, which can also increase our perceptions, temper, and assertiveness, blocking the flow of Divine logic.

Fear is the earth-bound energy that stops us from achieving, doing, living, believing, or remembering love. The Divine feminine, which is the right side of our body, is also off-balance when it is controlled by fear. The flow of our spirituality, compassion, and ability to move past trauma and pain takes a backseat, while fear swells, internally blocking us from receiving the energetic flow of Divine love. We may find ourselves separated from religion and community to the point where we question the existence of God.

Temptation and Challenge

Fear has many names: some refer to it as "evil," "the devil," or "Satan." The Divine has shown me that for most souls fear makes its first appearance in childhood, usually between the ages of four and six—although for some, fear does not arrive until later in life.

Fear enters our lives to challenge us through the temptation to give in or to give up. We need this challenge because our souls chose to come into this life to achieve and learn. Our lessons are the goals our souls set in place before we came into human form. Our souls desire evolution, expansion, and growing closer to God. These challenges are meant to propel us forward to our highest good, not keep us stuck in the past!

That is why we have chosen to live our life: to experience lessons, temptations, pains, and relationships. We are here not to be stopped by them but to see God's presence within them. We are called to choose love again and again, even within the moments of our greatest suffering.

God has endless love for us. God does not create temptation, evil, pain or suffering; fear is the one that does that. Fear is earth-bound energy and can transfer from person to person. It also has the ability to grow and multiply, as does love. Fear, when left unattended or unhealed, becomes bitterness, anger, hate, jealousy, resentment, and eventually can turn into evil.

God has provided us with many tools to resist fear and the energy that causes pain, isolation, and misery. Those gifts are: faith, hope, prayer, grace, forgiveness, compassion, sympathy, humility, respect, patience, and the greatest of all, love. But love is the first thing we learn to forget. It's hard to believe, but it is true. We are born with pure love, but it begins to fade through our exposure to other viewpoints from our family, friends, and others. Their fears slip in and begin manipulating our thoughts. One fear-based thought is planted within our mind and in that instant, love is forgotten. That is the moment when Shmego is born. One fearful thought pattern that has been passed down by another leads to our unbalanced ego.

Don't misunderstand me here: we need a healthy ego. Ego is our Divine masculine side, which is made up of healthy and balancing energy that supports our logic and journey in learning and growing in this life. But when corrupted by fear, ego and our Divine masculine become blocked—or worse, they grow into toxic energy, and we become overly analytical.

The Angels guided me to put an actual name on this energy to better teach me, and now others, how to best identify it: Shmego. The thing to understand is that Shmego is all ours. He knows us inside and out, along with all our weaknesses, doubts, guilt, pains and challenges, and he uses them to manipulate us. Shmego will have us believe the worst is true. He will have us become a victim of our own life while blaming, shaming, and framing other people for circumstances we don't like.

When this harmful energy grows and multiplies, our thoughts turn our healthy state of being into an unbalanced, open playing field for illness, disease, misery, and relationship destruction. Our life, as my older daughter says, becomes a "hot freakin' mess."

But we needn't worry, because we are not alone in that mess. The people who challenge us are also a hot mess. The family member who hurt us, the teacher who told us negative stuff, the doctor who took our hope away, that former friend who hurt us, the bully who picked on us, our parents, our families, our spouses—they are all a *hot freakin' mess*!

This is because evil's propaganda is an energetic earth-bound energy which is easily transmitted to others. It is also an energy that is effortless to pick up. For the most part, people don't understand that their personal energy matters to the well-being of the entire planet.

Our thoughts become our reality, our suffering lingers, life gets harder, and nothing seems to improve when Shmego rules our lives. This is why we must take inventory of our thoughts as often as possible, checking in to see if they are fear-based or love-based! This simple check-in is easy to do and will provide us with miracle moments infused with love.

The reason we don't fully understand how fear energy is transmitted person-to-person is that the human race as a whole has chosen to go it alone. This means faith and spirituality are not the norm for us. So many have turned away from religion and closed off their connection for one reason or another. But, my friend, this is not about religion; rather, it is about connecting to God. Although I attend church regularly with my family, I also believe in the importance of a daily connection to God through prayer and meditation. It's about calling your deity by name and, if need be, leaving religion out of the mix. There are countless ways to connect to God; don't let your relationship with Him suffer because of a manmade religion. The Angels say we should think of religion as a place of worship where there are four walls that humans have built to house their belief system and honor God, but the roof is meant to be open to allow the truth and light of Heaven in. Opening our mind and body to God will only improve our lives. Shutting out His love will leave us feeling like we are stranded in a storm.

The Five Fears

With a large portion of society spewing their feelings, opinions and moods on the news, social media and across the web, our planet has become a giant spinning sphere of terror. To begin to heal the planet of all this discharged negative energy, each and every soul alive needs to become aware of and accountable for their own fears. Accountability for our thoughts, actions and reactions is the first step in beginning the massive cleanup that is needed to heal the world. It is up to us to heal our own energy. Taking time to learn, grow, and heal will support us and others in the cleanup. Remember we have the power and tools to call the darkness out. We can be the light and love we need. We can stop, drop, and pray to cleanse our corner of the planet.

Awareness is required if we want to participate in the massive energetic healing of our planet. Therefore, be on the lookout for evil's temptation and warning signs. They are easy to spot once we know the five fears that challenge our commitment to God's love. The ***"five fears"*** are ***Desire***, ***Doubt***, ***Deception***, ***Destruction***, and ***Disloyalty***.

1. ***Desire*** is the strong feeling of wanting or wishing for something. In a fear state of mind, one would be drawn to desire what another human has or is. Desire therefore has a jealous energy attached to it. When we desire something or someone that is not aligned with our energy, we go against ourselves and God.

2. ***Doubt*** is an uncertainty. Acting from doubt means going without faith, without God. When doubt's voice is louder than love's voice, we are going against our own truths and pushing aside what God has intended for us. To be clear, doubt is different from contemplation. When we need time to mull something over, we can choose to examine all angles of the situation before making a decision.

3. ***Deception*** is the act of deceiving or lying. Whether we're deceiving ourselves or others, deception comes from the voice of fear. Half-truths, little white lies, or full-blown avoidance of our truths is and always will be the wedge that keeps us from experiencing love. Fear wants us to stay in this false state of living, a controlled state where one deception builds off another until love can no longer be seen or felt. Our loneliness and isolation are fear's victory.

4. ***Destruction*** is the action of causing damage to something to the point that it no longer exists. Breaking apart, causing harm, being the victim, and shutting out people is how fear wields its power to control us. We know love is absent when we have walked away from one or many relationships before healing them.

5. ***Disloyalty*** is the quality of not being loyal. When we are not honoring love and are corrupted by fear, our ego becomes overinflated in an unbalanced state. Our belief in God and love is challenged or closed off. Our faith has fallen, and we no longer trust others or our own intuition.

When we choose love over fear, it matters. Each and every time we change our fear thoughts over to love thoughts, it's a miracle. When we pray and invite God into our moment, it matters. When we forgive, well, that matters even more. When we let go, we heal one little energy droplet in our fear dumping ground. When we stop judging and open our heart to compassion, this matters too. For when we see others through the eyes of compassion, we are connecting to their God-spark, the truth of who they are. We are choosing to see them in love.

Let's chat a bit about the God-spark that is within us. This spark is also referred to as the seat of the soul, life force energy, the soul, breath of God and/or the Holy Spirit within. The Angels refer to our God-spark as the core of who we are. Our God-spark is what makes us who we are. It's God and us together. Only when we choose to ignore God, distancing ourselves from him, do our energies separate. Yes, we still carry on living and breathing, but we do so alone, without love as our guidepost. Some choose to deny God completely and go through life as atheists or with a science-based belief system. There is no right or wrong here, but there is a denial of original love.

When people make the choice to live disconnected from God and from original love, their life becomes complicated with the overgrowth of egotistical thoughts. Remember: logic is the Divine masculine energy and aids us in keeping a steady balance in the here and now. When ego is off-balance, faith begins to fade. Without faith, the ego makes way for fear to stomp out love. This is when Shmego takes over and searches for proof, wanting facts and forming opinions that, in turn, form walls of denial that keep love from reaching the heart. Knowledge and fact searching are addictions that can become the block that stops Divine love from entering our lives.

When fear becomes an addiction, it can be seen and felt miles away. It can also look different on someone other than yourself. We may feel their energy, see it, or even hear their negative tones spewing out of their mouths. Remember, this is because that constant terror speaks a language of its own, based on the five fears (desire, doubt, deception, destruction, and disloyalty).

A Legacy of Angst

Fear can work within us, and even carry through generations. I was able to see this in action when three sisters came to see me after their father passed away. Although there were five sisters in total, two remained at home because the family had been torn apart by their father's anger, fear, and grief. The sisters had been young adults when they lost their mother. For many years before and since, they had been caught up in the drama of their father's controlling words and narcissistic tendencies, aspects that only increased when their mother passed away. Their father manipulated one daughter at a time, slowly turning them against each other as they competed for his affections and tainted love. Then he passed on, leaving a difficult legacy for his daughters to untangle. They split into two teams; the three sisters who came to me composed one of these teams.

This form of control is dangerous for both parties. The three sisters knew they had to work through the memories to heal the wounds their father left behind. In order to heal the pain of him dangling his so-called love just out of reach, each sister would have to find her way to self-love and compassion. Only when she arrived in that space could each one begin to forgive. This type of pain can stay with us for a lifetime, or until we free ourselves from the burden of another person's misery. For the father, on the other hand, his healing would need to be done in Heaven. This is entirely possible, because the soul's work in Heaven is a continuum of the life on Earth, only without the fear.

During the reading, the sisters' mother came through first. Then the sisters sat in awe as I relayed how their father arrived with his head down, which is my sign for sorrow and shame. He spoke to his daughters one by one, apologizing for specific incidents that took place when he was alive.

As he released his sorrows, he also took responsibility for the pain he had inflicted.

Their father said things that many other souls do when they come through during readings: that he was sorry, and that he did not know the pain he had caused during his time on Earth. It often isn't until souls transition at death that they become aware of the pain they caused. Each of us goes through a purification, passing from the fear from our human life to the infinite love of our heavenly soul, which heals the past and opens a new celestial view of our years spent on Earth. This is how the soul can offer another the Divine grace of apology. Through their interaction with their father, the sisters healed much of the pain his fear had caused and were able to move forward with love.

The point of sharing the insights into this personal reading, as well as the other readings I've included in this book, is to spark a healing within us. The Angels show that when we connect with a message, even if it is for another person, our heart will open. This opening sparks an energetic chain of events, all of which lead toward healing.

Most people dismiss the importance of healing both our past and present life circumstances. But our souls are calling us to address the experiences that bind us to pain, suffering or unforgiveness, and the fear they leave behind.

Exercise

Let's look at our experiences from the viewpoint of fear, and then once again from the viewpoint of love.

Healing Stages from the Viewpoints of Love and Fear:

Think of a past event while considering the point of view you have taken as you remember it.

- **Love view:** We connect with a feeling inside of our being that comes from the signs or messages Spirit is sharing with us, such as: *You are beautiful, important, and meant to be here.*

vs Fear view: We judge these signs and messages, shut down, or even deny the connection being made, such as: *You are unworthy, unlovable, broken, and in need of fixing.*

- **Love view:** Our heart center opens. Love begins flowing.
  vs Fear view: Our mind starts chattering with fearful thoughts.

- **Love view:** Compassion arises. We feel warmth. Goose bumps may appear.
  vs Fear view: Judgments flood in, we feel angry or self-righteous. Our body is tense.

- **Love view:** A memory comes into our mind and warms our heart.
  vs Fear view: We think of our past and current life situations and victimhood rises.

- **Love view:** An emotional connection begins, tears or other forms of energy begin to release.
  vs Fear view: Our voice needs to be heard, so we begin stating our feelings, opinions, and beliefs—the "me, me, me, I, I, I" syndrome.

- **Love view:** We begin to feel lighter even freer than before. A healing that we were not fully aware of has taken place.
  vs Fear view: Our anger takes over, and we swoosh the messages to the side in full disbelief.

Journal Prompts:

After completing the exercise, use the following prompts to write about your experience in your journal.

- How can a different viewpoint allow you to reframe your past?
- What life circumstances are you willing to see in a different light?
- What other impressions did you receive from this exercise?

Fear's Contagion

Divine love flows when Spirit brings a group of people together for a reading in person, or even within a book. We can trust that the healing that is meant for us will come. There are mystical ways the Divine will weave the miracle of love and healing in our life. When we are open to receiving, the miracle moment arrives, my friend. This is because we are agreeing to invite the energetic love in.

Did you know that most people don't know that they are picking up fear energy and reacting to it? Well, it's a fact, Jack! Here is the down low, the Angel insider facts: when we see or feel someone's fear, we can inadvertently take that fear on without being aware of it. We then begin to react to that sponged-up fear. All of a sudden, without warning, our reactions are bigger than we are. Our feelings and emotions get con-jumbled up. In come frustrations that slowly morph into judgments; then manipulation comes into play. Manipulation tugs at us to help prove our point and stand our ground. Maybe even a little anger floats in and fires us up, and we end up responding in a fearful, mean tone. Or maybe denial comes in. We deny love, and in doing that, we deny our ability to speak and feel our soul's truths. Instead, we speak the other person's fears; we aid them by joining their victimhood, ranting and raving with them over injustices that fear insists are happening. That's a whole bunch of crazy going on! Right? And it all happened because fear played us! When aligned with our Soul Self, the energy of others and the injustices become mirrors that reflect the greater lesson at play.

The truth is that God does not want us to live in or with evil's misleading energy of fear; He would much rather that we choose love in the moment. Again, this is where our free will and life's lessons and tests are challenging us to learn, grow, and remember love. Choosing love will change our life instantaneously. We may doubt this truth because it is in our human nature to complicate things. The fact of the matter is that here on Earth we have the concept of time, and with time come restraints that complicate how we live and how we make our decisions. Our existence here on Earth comes not only with our soul's journey, our human conditioning, and the challenges fear places before us, but also with limited time. The Angels also say that our choice is simple and uncomplicated. All we need to do is choose love and stay in the present moment.

The truth is that we are more powerful than our thoughts. Our Shmego guy sends us thoughts that will have us believe that we are not powerful in any way. That's the bull-crap lie Shmego's negative tone wants us to believe. But in fact, we are love. Our souls are now and have always been connected to God. The connection is readily available for us to invite His Divine flow into our life. With our permission, we can heal the separation that is keeping us from living our soul's truth.

The Interplay of Faith, Hope and Love

Faith, hope and love—the gifts of God—are given through the Holy Spirit. They are gifted to us for our highest good. The gift of faith helps us let go and let God. The gift of hope is the energy that comforts, holds, and supports us. The gift of love, which is the greatest of all, can sustain us.

Through the gifts of faith and hope, love is the supporting factor. Without love, we will not experience the benefits of faith or hope, but with it, we can experience their bountiful graces. Faith and hope can be held as long as we require them. For instance, faith in God is held with our love for a lifetime. On the other hand, when we hold faith in a prayer, it is shorter term; that faith lasts until the prayer is answered or comes to fruition, but it is still held in love. Hope works the same way. We can hold hope for a positive outcome. While we do, love supports our hope, and when the positive outcome comes to fruition, our hope naturally fades away because it is no longer needed. Regardless, love remains.

Father Al, whom I spoke of earlier, taught through his great faith, extensive knowledge, and deep love for God. During an intimate family mass at my home several years ago, he shared a sermon that still replays in my mind. Father Al explained the energies of faith, hope, and love to my family during

our private mass. He said that when we hold faith in our heart, we support it with love, and when the faith fades, the love remains. The same is true when we hold hope for something or someone: again, our hope is supported by love. When what we've hope for comes, hope fades away, and what remains is love.

He used my daughter as an example. Her husband was deployed in Afghanistan. Of course, it was a tense and frightening situation—plus, they had a small baby at home. My daughter desperately hoped that her husband would arrive home in time for their daughter's baptism. She held this hope with love. He did return in time and her hope naturally faded away, leaving only her love remaining. Similarly, as her parents, we held faith and prayer for his safe return home from Afghanistan. Our faith naturally faded when he came home, and love remained.

Love is the one constant in all the universe. At any given moment we can stop what we are doing, breathe in, and connect to love simply by setting our intention to do so. We will find that when we choose love, it supports us, stands by us, and embraces us. Love gives us hope when we have none. Love reminds us that our faith can and will begin to erase the sadness, loneliness, isolation, anger, resentments, pains, hurts, sufferings, and emptiness we carry. Love will never leave us. Remember, it is evil's nature to send us thoughts that trick us into believing love has been taken from us. But the truth of love is that once it is given, it cannot be taken away. Love has been imprinted into every living being for our highest good; therefore, we have always had Divine love within us, and we will have it forevermore.

We are made of love. Love is creation. Love sustains our souls, helps us endure the darkest times, and remains steady and true all the while. Love tells us that anything chosen from love and with love is possible.

"Love's greatest gift is its ability to make everything it touches sacred."

— *BARBARA DE ANGELIS*

Love is universally available to each and every soul. Love, like God, doesn't conform into one belief system, religion, or idol. Love is beyond that which we see. It is eternal, as is God. God is love and love is God, infinite. And because God has gifted us free will, we can choose to invite Divine love and wisdom into our lives. Love can be our greatest asset in life. The corrupted energies of the masculine and feminine, held up by fearful ego and drenched with lies, block love's flow; these are what stop truth and all that is good from coming into our lives. But it's up to us to heal this. We do not have to wait for death to become the loving souls we are meant to be in this life! Now is the exact moment for us to cherish our loved ones, to forgive others and our past, to tell our family and friends we love them, to clean up our thoughts and stand with faith, hope, and love. This is how we can honor our highest good.

Chapter Five

CHAPTER FIVE

Our Life Path

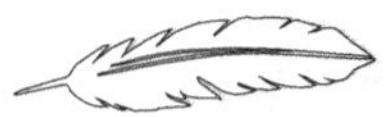

"You are on a soulful path that asks you to step into the greatest version of yourself. It is a sacred gift to shine your brightest light, not just in your moments of glory but each day."

— DEBBIE FORD

Our life path is unique to us. When a soul is preparing to leave this Earth, it has a destined route to take. The route is chosen by the soul and by God; the life mapping takes place before the soul is born. There are destined outcomes set in motion as the soul moves through life on the path it has chosen. That said, destiny is not a fated outcome or a one-way event.

Some say that the outcome of life is chosen by God, and that when God is ready for us, He will call us home. People may also say that a particular outcome was destined to happen. These are scenarios of a limited thought system. Love tells us that it is Shmego who keeps us from fully embracing the deeper connection to destiny. When we are out of our soul's alignment, which is the vertical connection to our higher Soul Self we spoke about in chapter one, we will find ourselves obscuring, dismissing, or ignoring our destiny.

> *"Every situation, properly perceived, becomes an opportunity to heal."*
> — *A COURSE IN MIRACLES*

Changing Destiny

The truth, as the Angels show me, is that our destined life can have many outcomes, not just one path. That is where our limited thinking comes into play. Destiny is predesigned, yet not written in stone. This is why it is a dangerous business to try and map out our lives and see into the future. We may have a desire to know our fate, but remember God has given us free will, which means our future cannot be fully predicted. Keep in mind that while our destiny is always at play and so, my friend, are our choices: to live with love or to follow fear's deceptions. Let's break this down a bit further to better illuminate how there are only fear and love. We can see this easily by breaking down our choices into action words. Fear actions come with words such as "denial," "avoidance," and "procrastination." If we change the tone, thoughts, and actions over to love, then *denial* becomes *acceptance*; *avoidance* becomes *meditative*; and *procrastination* becomes *restful*.

In this way, our life's route is in our hands. What's more, while bad things do happen to good people, good people also make mistakes. It's just a matter of removing fear to see the truth. Lessons that challenge us can be the stopping point of our life or the pathway for our greatest growth.

Take the reading I did with Kalyn as the perfect example of how one's preconceived notion of destiny can be shifted, healed, and changed. When Kalyn first came for her reading, the Angels impressed me with the message that she had been sexually abused. The instant she sat down, I heard the message of abuse loud and clear. I also knew from the energy that surrounded her that she was in a very low place. I could feel her sadness within my mind and body, which led me to know that I needed to broach the subject carefully. At first I thought the reading was going to be about the trauma that was inflicted on her, but then suddenly the messages shifted in a completely different direction. The Angels were impressing the tone of suicide and drugs.

A young man stepped forward from the veil and spoke of overdosing and conveyed the taste of toxins and the feeling of being poisoned, which is my sign of an accidental overdose. He claimed Kalyn as his sister and stood by her side with his hand on her shoulder. Kalyn confirmed this to be her half brother who had overdosed years earlier. Her brother spoke of his addiction and wanted Kalyn to know that he had not planned on taking his life; rather, his untimely death was a result of his lack of self-respect. He said that Kalyn believed that she, too, would find death in a similar manner. Her brother also began impressing the feeling of inappropriate behavior which caused a sick feeling within my stomach. I shared with Kalyn what her brother was showing me. What the Angels showed me next was that the sexual misconduct I had felt in the beginning of the reading was actually not about her being abused by another, but rather about the fact that Kalyn was abusing her own body. The impressions came to me of self-inflicted pain, with Kalyn cutting herself and having addictions to both sex and drugs. Her brother also spoke about the suicidal thoughts that she was replaying over and over in her mind.

Emotional and crying, Kalyn confirmed her brother's messages as she began to share all of the negative decisions she had been making. Kalyn shared that she believed that her brother had died from an overdose and that she would eventually too. She went on to say that her father had also made statements about her passing just like her brother. Kalyn said she had been wanting to ask for help but did not know where to go. Another message came to me, saying I needed to speak about her being an empath. This came as a feeling inside my body through a heightening of my senses. The Angels have taught me through many readings that this is my sign to begin asking the empath questions. I began the series of questions and confirmed that she was indeed an empath. Then we spoke about her brother's addiction and what it felt like to me and how she, too, was feeling the energy of it inside her body. Kalyn began to uncover that she was feeling the suffering of her brother and acknowledged that it was confusing to her. This made it challenging for her to distinguish between her own feelings and that of her deceased brother. We spoke about ways for her to regain balance within her body while disconnecting from the energy of her brother's overdose. We also talked about basic tools for her to use to feel her own energy and the ways she could clear and balance herself each and every day.

Kalyn left feeling empowered by knowing how to start creating her own healthy support system using therapy, her new tools and conversations with her mother. Her brother also reassured Kalyn that she had his support from Heaven—that he and his love were always available to her.

Beyond the reading itself, it was also a miracle moment that brought Kalyn and me together in the first place. I met her when my husband and I went out for dinner one night; she was our waitress. I normally don't receive messages from Spirit when I am "off duty" but that night, Spirit nudged and gently pushed me to speak up—and it has become my practice to listen when Spirit urges me to do something. I found myself telling Kalyn about the work I do and how I communicate with Angels and loved ones in Heaven. Each time she came back to our table, we spoke about the pain that she was living with, while my hubby sat and smiled at the beautiful connection unfolding before him. By the time the check came, I knew that there was far more to Kalyn's story then we had the time to discuss during our meal. Not fully knowing why, I offered her my business card and invited her to come for a reading when and if she was ready. I did, however, trust Spirit's guidance. Now I know that it saved this young girl from the painful path she was on, wherein she was convinced that she, too, was destined to die of an overdose.

The Angels show me that while God does have a plan for us, it is intertwined with the path we have chosen to experience in this life. God also says that we are invaluable souls with endless choices to make. It's up to us to fulfill the reason we have been born. Your reason is unique to you; your lessons, value system, and choices are all yours.

Our Soul's Journey

God will not interfere with our soul's journey to learn and grow. He will support us, love us, and guide us, especially when we have lost our way. God is the one who most people blame for a life gone astray, an untimely death, an act of evil, and so many other life events—but God is not to blame: fear is. Fear turns the mind against truth. And because the mind is a sponge for learning, it can also be the breeding ground for untruth. That is fear doing the work of evil.

Because each soul will come into life for a specific reason, that soul will choose a community of other souls to work with in order to help support each other during their time together. It is true that we choose our family. Those early relationships are in place to lay the foundation for your life lessons and journey. Collectively, souls will also come together in life to experience lessons on a larger level. Take Liza, for example, whom I met at a group reading.

It is common for souls to come through as I meditate and prepare for readings, and this night was typical in that way; even before I left my home and we settled in for the evening's event, I was receiving messages from the departed souls connected to the living people I had yet to meet. One female soul that came through earlier in that day was impressing upon me a deep emotional pain that had been passed on and carried down through her family. She also gave my body the feeling of depression and anxiety. I felt the anxiety within my chest area. I couldn't seem to take a deep breath and the depression was intense, as if all hope had been separated out and only a lack of joy remained.

I began the evening's group reading with my normal introduction about who I am and how I work. I then went around the room to get each person's name and answer any questions they had before leading the group in a guided meditation.

As soon as this group took their seats, Spirit flooded my body and mind with even stronger anxiety and suicidal tones than the ones it had impressed within my body earlier in the day. Spirit then brought my attention to a woman seated on the sofa. I could see the energy of her aura was vibrating at a low frequency and was a brownish color, which I took to mean that her energy centers were blocked with fear.

Spirit runs the show during events such as this one, so where my attention is drawn is where I begin the readings. This is how I came to meet Liza. Her grandmother's soul stepped forward and shared personal details of their relationship. As Liza's grandmother continued, she shared the impression that Liza was filled with anxiety that was depleting her energy. Her departed grandmother spoke of the disconnection from the Divine and then led me to see that Liza's fourteen-year-old daughter had attempted suicide. Liza sobbed, confirming the message by nodding her head. The Angels guided me to see with my third eye that Liza was disconnected from religion, and that this disconnection had harmed her relationship with God. This appears around the person as a broken strand of light illuminating from the crown of the head upward to Heaven. Her grandmother then shared that Liza and her parents' relationship had been closed off due to their different views on religion. I gently shared this information with Liza as the Angels guided me with soft and loving words that would spark hope and faith to reach Liza's heart.

The effect of this reading was profound. At the end of the night, Liza came over to me and asked if I could help her further. We talked for a bit, and I gave her my contact information to use when she was ready. After a couple of weeks, Liza set up a private appointment for herself and another for her daughter, Jenna.

Jenna's first reading was emotional for both of us. She sat across from me on the sofa with her head down, her arms crossed, and a closed-off attitude. I said a prayer and began the reading.

When Spirit impresses in me the energy of suicidal thoughts, I am also impressed with whether this suicidal energy belongs to the person I am reading or if they have energetically picked up these thoughts and feelings from someone else. Spirit shared that Jenna is an empath and that though she had attempted suicide, the energy did not originate from inside her body. Rather, Jenna had inadvertently absorbed the suicidal energy from another. I was shown in my mind that Jenna was also cutting herself to "feel," as well as manipulating others in order to create friendships.

I wasn't surprised; the Angels have shown me that it is not uncommon for sensitive souls and/or empaths to cause harm to their bodies. They do this because they are unaware that they are picking up and absorbing others' energy, and this form of pain is a way to "feel" their own energy. Jenna was clearly a strong empath, and she was at a very tender moment in her development.

Spirit had me use a direct tone, going straight to the point without messing around so that Jenna would know I knew the truth. We spoke openly about her tendencies to manipulate people and the lies that were causing pain, both in her peer relationships and within her family. Jenna's departed great-grandmother came through and spoke about how Jenna was verbally abusive to her mother and was actually causing harm to herself as a way to punish others when she wasn't able to get her own way. I gave her tools to use right away that would help her regain her connection to herself and release the energy of others.

Spirit then shared that Jenna is a talented artist and her art would be a large part of the pathway for her return to self. Jenna confirmed she could paint and draw but no longer had the time or the desire to do it. We spoke about the importance of finding time for her self-discovery through her talents. I explained how using her artistic talents would balance her energy and her gifts.

By the end of the session, Jenna was sitting with her arms by her side, smiling and willing to take part in her healing.

I have since met with Liza and Jenna several times over the course of two years. While they have moved forward, they have also experienced setbacks and had to work through painful past events. Liza, as she healed her separation from religion and began releasing and forgiving her parents, found that her relationship with her husband began to improve. She began practicing small acts of self-love, opened her spirituality, and welcomed God back into her life. True healing comes when we agree to it on a mind, body, and soul level. Liza found that self-loathing was keeping her from her truths and personal power. She had unknowingly held the pain of her past closely and believed she had no power to change her life or help her daughter.

Jenna learned to address the manipulative energy she used to control others with fear. Because Jenna could feel her mother's weakened state of energy, she caused chaos in order to gain love and attention. She also didn't know how to ground her spiritual talents with creativity and self-care. All this led to her feeling hopeless about her future. Today, Jenna is a happy, self-assured young woman who creates art to express her feelings. Her relationship with Liza is dramatically improved, and she is planning for college.

While our lessons and life events may be painful for us to go through, they are also invitations to live in our greatness. By healing a generational wound or a lineage of suffering, we are aligning to our individual purpose as well as to the greater generational purpose of our family's collective healing.

Returning to Love

"Love created me like itself.... Love holds no grievances."

— *A COURSE IN MIRACLES*

The return to love can be very challenging. Shmego will try his best to hold us in the past. We may sense this tug of war; with each step we take toward the truth of love, Shmego will fight to pull us back into the old memories, stories, and justifications that fuel fear. Our job is to keep looking forward, take the next step toward truth and love, and to call Shmego out as the lying thief that he is! In time, we will find, although the struggle is real, the "you work" that we put in pales in comparison to the benefits we will reap as we begin to live a life centered in love and authenticity, connected to Divine truth.

If you are like me, you may have experienced anxiety or depression at some point in your life. You may have taken or currently be taking medication for these ailments. I understand this completely and do not judge it. Yet I often find that these situations are not only chemical; there is often a spiritual component, and healing the condition starts with forgiveness.

Shedding the past with compassion for ourselves and offering forgiveness and compassion to the ones who hurt us is part of our healing. Forgiveness is a pivotal action to our healing. Letting go is the gift we give ourselves and others. Self-love reminds us that God has our back and that the past can be our greatest gift—a stepping stone that lays the foundation to a bright and shiny now.

There is a formula I would like to share, one that I tell my clients when they are suffering by not letting go of the past: "Depression comes from living in the past; anxiety comes from living in the future; but love is in the present." This means love is our gift of being in this moment. That is why being in the now is called the "present"—it's a gift we give ourselves! I also like to share with my clients that, while a loved one may have caused them great pain in life, a purification happens for each living soul when they cross to the other side of the veil. If that soul has passed out of its body, it has grown significantly.

Let me explain a little more about purification.

The purification process that we go through before entering Heaven is a removal of any and all earth-bound fear energy that the soul has accumulated during life on Earth, thus returning the soul to original love. In Heaven, there is an absence of both fear and time. There is only *love*. Fear, as we have discussed throughout this book, is an earth-bound energy that attaches itself to many aspects of our lives.

Some souls will begin to purify here on Earth. This purification can look like suffering to the human eye. What the Angels have shown me is that what we might see as someone's suffering as they go through the dying process is actually their soul purifying. The purification is a cleansing of the earth-bound fear that has accumulated over the lifetime, and each soul has a unique type of purification to go through. A soul can choose to begin to purify here on Earth in order to expand and learn valuable lessons. The soul can also purify here in order to release and heal a karmic pattern. This is not a punishment by God, but rather a pathway to move closer to God in healing energy and learning from their soul experiences.

When souls cross over, they purify by leaving all fear behind them so that by the time they reach Heaven, only love remains. The memory stays, but the fear leaves. That is how a soul will come through in a reading with a love tone, even if they caused great pain to themselves and to others during their life here on Earth.

Forgiveness is given to all souls who align with God. When we enter Heaven through those pearly gates we have heard about, when we stand before God's kingdom, we are welcomed with love, forgiveness, and eternal peace. Our loved ones welcome us, as do the hierarchy of celestial beings of God's love. Heaven welcomes us with open arms of unconditional love, wisdom, and grace as we leave our human form. Every soul is welcomed and will continue its journey from the point when it left the physical body in a type of heavenly school. The soul's life is illuminated in the reflections of Earth without the influence of fears involvement. The loved ones I've spoken to say that the colors in Heaven are brighter, almost as if they are cleaner than we've seen them. The essence of Heaven is on Earth.

Each soul will continue to learn and expand upon the lessons of its life experiences. Because Heaven has no boundaries, the souls are much more aware that they are interconnected than they are here. That means no personal agendas, broken relationships, jealousy, lying, manipulation, or cheating. As the soul heals, it can move to a higher plane of existence. The soul can choose to either have another physical human life experience, thus expanding and deepening the current lesson, or expand on to a new soul lesson there in Heaven. When a soul incarnates, it sets in motion a well-mapped plan to work collectively with other souls on larger lessons.

The Angels have said that the timing in Heaven is obsolete, meaning there is no measure of when. They say a soul incarnation happens when God determines. This can be immediately after passing or can take several human life cycles. The reason and timing depend on the soul's journey. That is how our life experiences can be taken with us and carried into a new life. These experiences can display themselves as a feeling of familiarity, such as when we have the sense of already knowing a place, event, or person before we technically have reason to. The soul is infinite, so experiences and people come into our life to support our soul's journey. Although they may challenge us, hurt us, or anger us, they are there to teach us. That is the journey of the soul: to support each other in ways we can't fully understand.

"The joy is always in the journey and when you get that, then it just does not matter very much at all where you are currently standing."

— *ABRAHAM HICKS*

Relationships That Challenge Us

Challenging relationships are mirrors for our growth. Though we won't always like every person we meet, there are those challenging people that will particularly bug us or get under our skin. The reason they are there for us, and us for them, is that God has given us mirrors to help us know ourselves. The reflection we see when looking at the people who challenge us carries a message or lesson to help expand our growth. It is within the challenge that we can see this message—we need only to slow our propensity to anger and open to compassion instead. It is when we allow love to flow through us that we are able to see a connection in another's eyes, and this connection informs us about the lesson that is now available for us to learn. Learning this lesson is a healing that shifts our lives in ways that are bigger and far more valuable than we could ever imagine.

These challenging relationships often carry old fear because, while there is no fear between lifetimes, it can certainly be carried from one life form to another. This can often look like an irrational behavior or even a phobia of something. Although the life experience will be different, our original soul's lessons will repeat until they are healed. Lessons can seem painful, annoying, and downright senseless, but they are our soul's pathway to enlightenment.

Enlightenment is achieved when our soul has healed from the pain learned through our lessons and when we live life purely in alignment with God.

"We human beings don't realize how great God is. He has given us an extraordinary brain and a sensitive loving heart. He has blessed us with two lips to talk and express our feelings, two eyes which see a world of colours and beauty, two feet which walk on the road of life, two hands to work for us, and two ears to hear the words of love. As I found with my

ear, no one knows how much power they have in their each and every organ until they lose one."

— MALALA YOUSAFZAI

Relationships that bring us to replay old behaviors, feel judged, become defensive or angry, and feel misunderstood are telltale signs that fear is tripping us up! Below is a love healing meditation that will guide you to heal a broken or challenging relationship or painful life experience.

Exercise

Try this meditation when you are challenged by a person or a situation—especially when you see fear begin to act.

Love Healing Meditation:

Sit upright or lie down with your spine straight.

Begin your cycle breathing, inhaling through your nose and exhaling through your mouth. Do several rounds of breathing and, when your body relaxes, move through the following steps.

With your next inhalation, bring your attention and your breath to the crown of your head. As you exhale, notice a glistening Divine light that flows from the Heavens above through your crown and into your body.

Bring your awareness and your breath to the center of your chest.

As you breathe into your heart center, notice the Divine light enter your heart and visualize a sparkly, emerald-green light swirling and filling your chest cavity. As you continue breathing into your heart center, the emerald-green light expands and fills your chest cavity.

In your mind, envision the person or event that you are working to heal. Imagine this reflection directly in front of you. With your next inhalation, connect with your heart center and the Divine emerald light as you send it outward, surrounding both you and the image.

Allow yourself time to release the connections that bind you to this pain. Feeling protected with Divine love, offer forgiveness, compassion, and love to your pain.

Stay embraced in this loving energy as the picture before you fades away. Then bow your head in reverence and reflect on the love that remains in its place.

When you are ready you can invite another healing forward, or you can invite the light back into your being as you rest here in this meditation for as long as you need.

Journal:

Write in your journal about how you are feeling and any experiences you had.

Seeing Life as a Soul Journey

Our life experiences enrich our soul's journey. Everything—the choices we make, the forgiveness we offer, the decisions we make—causes our soul to expand when done with love and with God at our side. The foundational gift God has given us to live our life, heal our pain, learn our lessons, ward off temptations and raise our vibration is: *Love.*

We can get a glimpse of how we can begin to take our power back and choose love through our action of forgiveness. We can also send our love, compassion, and forgiveness outward to the one who caused us pain. When we allow ourselves to see as our equal and our teacher the person who caused us pain, we are able to free our energy and theirs from being bound to the past.

When we commit to this, we begin to see life as a phase of our soul's journey. Individual events that cause us harm gain a greater context; they become part of a greater purification that culminates in our body's death. This purification, too, is merely a segment of our path. Understanding this helps to set us free.

Chapter Six

CHAPTER SIX

The Personal Moral Code

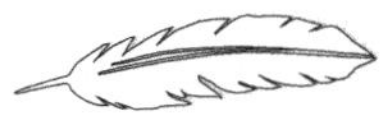

"The privilege of a lifetime is being who you are."

—*JOSEPH CAMPBELL*

Living out of alignment with our Soul Self will leave us depleted in ways we may not fully understand. The path of innocence, meaning the naïve choices of our actions taken without a connection to God, will set us up to follow a path of separation. Acts like becoming aware of our thoughts, feelings, resentments, anger, and stories, while seemingly appearing as singular occurrences, are choices that layer together energetically. Living apart from our soul truth—the truth that God and love are our soul's destiny—is the path of innocence, my friend, and in choosing this, we are setting the intention to go it alone. Our saving grace is when we're able to live by a higher moral code, one that is individual to each of us. This starts with intention. It is important to fully understand that our intention is one of our most powerful gifts and strongest assets; it's the king.

The Personal Moral Code (PMC)

The intention we hold behind our decisions carries the weight of our soul's moral code. We all have a personal moral code, or PMC, by which we live. The PMC is our soul's contract with God to live a love-based life wherein we dedicate ourselves to learning our specific and unique lessons. Just as we set the intention to follow a particular religion, set of moral beliefs or code of ethics, we also must set the intention to follow our PMC. The PMC of our soul is designed by God and is woven into our soul's journey. While there are moral codes that are in place for all humankind, such as the Ten Commandments, we also have our very own code to follow for our soul's well-being.

When our PMC is off, our choices go against love, and our soul's lessons become burdens we struggle to carry instead of opportunities for learning and growth. We all have at least one main life lesson that we've come here to learn.

For instance, one of my life lessons is to choose to self-love, and my PMC is compassion for self and others. Self-love holds the truth of my soul, while the denial of self-love hides my truths, opening the door for judgment to come in. What this means is that when I choose to go it alone, ignoring the gift of connection to Spirit, I am not supporting Divine truth; I am not inviting love to move with me. It is then that I self-doubt, self-loathe, and begin the cycle of disconnecting from my Soul Self. When that happens, I second-guess myself, feel terrible, my body aches, and I am lonely, even though I have a loving family and devoted spouse. I am also not able to see others with the compassion that they deserve, because I am judging them as well as myself. When I choose to go it alone, I isolate myself from love. Both my PMC and my intention are to live with compassion for myself and for others, and in doing so, I choose God. It is then that I begin living in alignment with my Soul Self, and only when I am actively doing that am I able to use my gifts and talents with ease to fulfill the purpose of why I am here.

Our PMC is activated by our intention moment by moment, choice by choice. When we make a conscious decision to go against our PMC, in essence we hurt our own soul.

Recognizing our life lesson can come into our awareness as we consistently practice meditation and do our "you work." I recommend a daily prayer and meditation practice of twenty minutes, followed by time to journal and reflect inward, as a path for growth, self-discovery, and healing. Praying is our personal way of connecting with God, asking for blessings for ourselves and others, showing gratitude and offering our love and devotion. Meditation is our personal space for hearing God's answers and guidance. One without the other leaves us feeling unsupported, but used in connection with each other, they become invaluable tools.

The exercise below can help you write down Spirit's guidance and the inner dialogue that comes to the surface during meditation.

Exercise

This exercise can help you get in touch with the life lessons you came here to learn, which will in turn inform your own PMC.

Life Lessons:

Look back over your past relationships, notice the common themes between them, as well as any similarities to your present relationships, and write them down.

For the next week, set your intention in prayer and meditation for your life lesson to come into your view. Spend time writing in your journal after each meditation. You can also add a daily prayer petition in your journal.

Journal Prompts:

After completing the exercise, use the following prompts to write about your experience in your journal.

- What is the most painful thing you've experienced in your life?
- When did this experience take place?

- List the people in both present and past relationships who challenged you.
- Do you have a pattern of repeating relationships with people? What is the pattern?
- Do you find yourself reliving similar challenges? What are those challenges?
- When you take a step back from the current pain you are experiencing, can you see its main cause?

To better help you discover more about your life lessons and PMC and support your journey, I've created resources for you on my website. See *believeangels.com*.

Going Against the PMC

Remember our souls are infinite, but they can still be harmed. The connection to our Soul Self frays energetically when we go against our PMC. Our soul connection will begin to actually weaken in our beings, slowly disconnecting us from Divine Source. We feel less and less like ourselves the more we go against our moral code and our soul's truth.

Jessica's story reflects how going against our PMC can send our lives off course.

When Jessica booked her appointment with me, she stated that she wanted the best of what I offered; she wanted to try every offering in one session. I knew it would be some combination of a mediumistic reading, a healing and angelic guidance, but like her, I had no idea what the session would hold.

When we met, I instantly began to see evidence of an off-balance life in her energy field. As she sat on the couch in my office, Jessica spoke about why she had come: She wanted healing and clarity around her business, which had once been booming but was now in a lull. As she spoke, I noticed the energy surrounding Jessica's throat had a weakness to it. The Angels began to indicate how she could get back on track, so I communicated this to her. But as I did, they also began to show me that she was not being truthful. I was led not to broach that subject with Jessica just yet.

As we continued on, it seemed that every message annoyed Jessica rather than soothed her, even when loved ones came through, such as deceased family members who addressed the alcoholic home in which she had grown up and her former business partner who had passed away from a cancer that he had not told her about. In most circumstances, these sorts of messages would be highly impactful. Some people have what I call a "no-no-no block," meaning they deflect the messages because their soul is not ready and open to receive them yet. Curiously, this was not the case with Jessica; rather, the messages had no value or merit for her because she wasn't being truthful with herself.

As we continued, Jessica started asking questions that seemed disconnected from the reading. I was taken aback and invited Spirit to assist me further. Then Spirit again impressed in my mind that she was lying and showed me the serpent, my sign for deceit, which I took to mean that it was time to address the issue with Jessica. When I looked her in the eye and asked her why the Angels kept showing me that she was lying, her face dropped and her eyes welled up with tears.

We sat for a few moments as the message sank in; I could see that her energy was weakened by the lies and by going against her moral code. She began to tell me that she was in an intimate relationship with a coworker, but she wasn't fully admitting to herself that it was indeed a relationship, and she was actively hiding it from the outside world. I was shown this was why her business and now her home life seemed to be in a perpetual "Groundhog Day" state, without growth or change, and why she was unable to receive the loving, healing messages her loved ones were sharing. She needed to hear that she was the one causing this pain in her own life.

Jessica's life lesson is to live and be truth. Her journey through life has challenged her to be truthful, and it has shown her this through the trouble she's faced in her relationships. The business partner who lied about his illness and the mother who covered up for the father's alcoholic behaviors provide two examples. Jessica's journey has presented plenty of reasons to not be the lies but the truth instead, and living in alignment with her PMC requires her to commit to a life of truth.

I explained to Jessica that in order for the messages to have the healing effect they are meant to have, she will have to continue to be open to love. This way, she will be able to learn from her experiences and the life lessons that come with them, instead of allowing them to burden her soul.

As Jessica's story indicates, the secret to finding our PMC is in getting to know our own strengths and weaknesses, and this requires being honest about our feelings and knowing the voice of Shmego. But it's not easy to connect to our deep-seated feelings and emotions, nor to the reason we are holding them inside our body. These emotions and feelings have likely been kept under lock and key for a long time, so they may not even make full sense to us when they arise.

The Body Remembers

The Angels want us to know that fear is the most common reason that our pain and suffering remains unhealed. We end up holding these memories in our bodies, which act as a type of storage unit for old, unprocessed fear. While it is true that we will hold loving memories inside our bodies as well, they are not harmful; their energy is light, bright, and airy. These loving memories remain part of our memory center and connect with our heart. This is why when we think of a happy memory, our brains trigger a response and send a signal for our heart to open. We feel lighter and brighter; our brains trigger receptors in the nervous system and that feel-good effect flows through the entire body.

So, how do we know if we are storing old and unhealthy memories? The evidence is similar to our happy memory response: there is a physical reaction within the body. Of course, to properly observe this reaction, we must be able to distinguish the voice of love from the voice of Shmego. But we also need to break down the barrier of fear around the memory we're holding within our body; we have to be willing to feel the raw edges of uneasiness that may arise. The raw edges are the feelings and emotions that magnetically draw our attention toward the negative aspects of the memory.

The confusion comes when fear kicks in and we go into fight or flight mode. This causes us to protect the memories that Shmego has tricked us into believing are accurate. When this happens, our hearts begin to beat faster, and we literally get the urge to fight, verbally or physically, or run away and not deal with what is happening. When we are afraid, we seek safety; it is a built-in mechanism for survival. Over time, when fear has replaced our thought system and memories, the blockages in our body grow and multiply. The longer love is kept away from these memories, the harder it is to uncover the fear that surrounds and blocks them.

We can see this in moments when pain suddenly sparks. These spark moments awaken the feelings, emotions, sensations, or rawness of our memories. This happens not to cause us to feel pain, but rather to invite an opportunity for healing into our life.

Because here's the truth: it is in the moment of raw uneasiness, discomfort, even anger, that we are able to witness our true power to forgive, to say we're sorry, and to rewrite the memory, infusing love into the fear. Then we can go back and look at our memory with new eyes. We can relive that particular moment in time, seeing where love was actually available to us and a lesson was presenting itself.

Each time we shed a part of a painful memory, we heal one energetic layer of fear. These layers take time and patience to heal. We may feel like we are done with looking over the same memory in our life, but then, all of a sudden, another spark moment comes, and we are once again transported back in time. Or we may live in complete denial that these memories actually exist within us. This sort of attitude is dangerous; it keeps us from seeing the root cause behind our physical ailments and the blocking points in our life. The limited mind will have us believe we can bury the past and it will have no bearing on our life in the present moment, but our minds expand when we can be in our higher Soul Self and witness our life in a new way: as a pathway of living with God and unconditional love.

Healing Evil

"Love is the bridge between you and everything."

— *RUMI*

Finding the viewpoint in Rumi's quote may be hard to do, especially if we have been the recipient of an act of wrongdoing or evil caused by another human soul. The Angels say that it is in these challenging life moments that our soul is being called to surrender to faith. We don't find forgiveness for the people who have hurt us; we do it for God and for the Source living within each of us.God does not cause the evil that grows on this planet; that is the action birthed from fear, and as I've noted, fear is not of God. Because fear is a heavy, earth-bound energy, it is easily transmitted from one human to another, and it can also easily be dismissed as separate from us. That is because fear is not of us; we are not born with it, but rather it is an earthly energy that we absorb into our body. Fear then attaches itself to our thoughts, and then begins the corruption of energy within our being. This tempting energy grabs hold of the soul, challenging the truth of love and pulling it downward, away from God. As we know, every soul has a destiny to learn and grow, moving closer to God. Yet we may not fully grasp the truth that each soul has an equal ability to do this.

Jesus says that fear is the energy of what we call Hell and is an earth-bound energy. And while every soul is a child of God, the souls that cause great harm to others do have a price to pay in eternity under God's judgment. Karma is the energy that all souls carry with them until the wrong deed is healed and transformed into love. Again, this is not God's way to punish souls but rather the soul's way of learning a valuable lesson that aids in the healing process.

The absence of love in one's life represents a disconnection with God. The simple truth is that acts of wrongdoing, or karmas, happen when a soul chooses fear over love. The Angels say that we form opinions early in our lives. Opinions based in love bond with our souls and cause us to act in ways that will restore any karmic energy our soul has been carrying. Opinions based in fear become a physical part of our being. This leaves a painful imprint in our bodies and causes us to act in ways that harm others and disrupt our soul's connection to God.

Restoring balance is part of our human journey, and that means healing fear is imperative. The problem is that we need God to do this and, for most of society, God is not in the forefront of daily life. Instead, fear energy draws us in, enticing us with false hope of something gained. When we give in to this, we end up losing the valuable time our soul needs to experience and expand in this life. Wasting time inevitably transforms into a fear-based addiction.

Fear addiction is a characteristic that the majority of humans possess. I shared my story of fear addiction at the beginning of this book, and in greater detail in *The Goddess You*. By choosing fear, I was denying my gifts and separating from my Goddess truths. I hope that sharing this view into my life will provide a mirror for others to witness how fear sneaks in, often before we even realize it is there and becomes a part of our daily life. The first step to healing addiction is admitting it exists. By connecting to the energy of our own addiction, we can begin to reverse the damage that addiction has had on our life. This can be an aha moment for us and a miracle moment in God's eyes. It is the beginning of healing evil, bringing us back to our Divine destiny and our PMC.

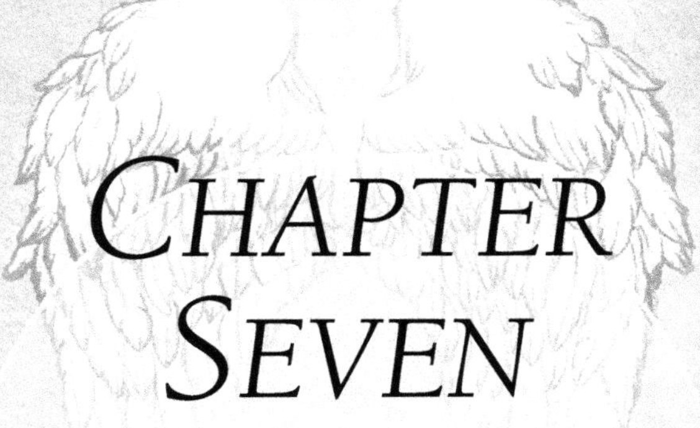

Chapter Seven

CHAPTER SEVEN

Gifts and Talents

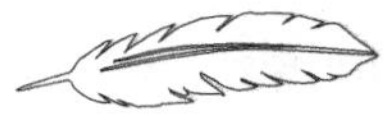

"Your talent is God's gift to you. What you do with it is your gift back to God."

— LEO BUSCAGLIA

Our gifts and talents are part of what makes us who we are. When we deny our truths, meaning our gifts and talents, we also deny God's love for us. Our souls have unique talents and gifts available to help us move along our life paths. Our talents are interwoven into our souls and are meant to enhance our gifts with action and expression of Divine love. I call the actions we take to use our talents while expressing God's love our *ings*—cooking, cleaning, painting, designing, creating, writing, running, snorkeling, and so forth.

Have you ever felt like you have no talents or that there is nothing special about you? Well, my friend, you are not alone in that painful thought pattern. The truth is that you are talented beyond the limited ideas that fear has set you up to believe. I know this simply because the Angels told me, and as I say Angels don't lie. This life we are living has a greater purpose. We are designed to succeed with love, to conquer fear, and shine our talents and gifts forward. Living our life's purpose is a scary feat, and it requires that our superhero Soul Self rise to the occasion. Our talents can aid us through our most challenging times by providing an outlet for our emotions and feelings to flow outward, while our gifts can comfort us by bringing the flow of Divine love inward, guiding and reassuring us to face our lessons with ease.

"There are different kinds of gifts, but the same Spirit distributes them."
— *CORINTHIANS 12:4 NIV*

Our Gifts Link Us to the Divine

God is always with us, in every situation. His love guides us through our challenges victoriously. In order to pass the test, we must first have a strong faith in place. Let's talk about those mundane feelings that arise from doing the same repetitive daily routines. They can be the reason we get bored and sidetracked, and ignore facing our challenges instead of taking the time to connect with our gifts and express them with love. By slowing ourselves down to connect our gifts with the task at hand, we can easily express ourselves and work through any resistance or challenge in our daily routine with Divine love.

Our gifts are the support system that connect us to the Divine. Everyone has talents and gifts that are unique to their soul and their soul's journey. Fully opening our gifts requires that we first be in alignment with our Soul Self; that's when passion, also known as love, leads us to our life's purpose!

Once we have cleared the pathway to our soul alignment by applying the twelve Goddess principles, we can begin to uncover our gifts and talents.

Most of us want to be able to use our gifts immediately, but we often don't take the necessary time to honor the process of doing the "you work" that is required to support keeping our gifts balanced and open. In contrast, what we actually experience are the lows of feeling drained of energy, and this inevitably causes us to welcome that Shmego guy back into our life. I've learned this crash-and-burn feeling firsthand, and that is why I want to save you the trouble of having to go backward! So there it is, my friend, in black and white: we have to do the "you work" to achieve what we want in life.

The Role of Pain

If you need even more inspiration to do the "you work," I suggest listening to Glennon Doyle Melton's SuperSoul Session, entitled "First the Pain, Then the Rising." It is awe-inspiring! I love how inspirational, funny, wise, and honest Glennon is about getting through the most challenging part of healing her pain.

Glennon also shares a poignant message about facing pain, not avoiding it, in her book *Love Warrior*:

Most of the messages we receive every day are from people selling easy buttons. Marketers need us to believe that our pain is a mistake that can be solved with their product ... *fix your hot loneliness with THIS*. So we consume and consume but it never works, because you can never get enough of what you don't need. The world tells us a story about our hot loneliness so that we'll buy their easy buttons forever. We accept this story as truth because we don't realize that their story is poison in our air. Our pain is not the poison: the lies about the pain are.[1]

She encourages us to not avoid the pain, explaining that not only do we need it but it was also meant for us. *Our pain is meant for us! Wow!* That may seem harsh, especially when we are facing challenges that are so hard. Here's the truth the Angels share: life is indeed hard. If we are experiencing turmoil, chaos, pain, illness, trauma, or any challenging life event, we are perfectly normal; we are like each and every soul on the planet. We all have our own pain to heal.

I know this to be true for myself, and I've witnessed it with my clients. If we try to just fix, outrun, cover or hide our pain, we will never find the relief our souls need. Avoiding our pain and our healing leaves us feeling depleted and unhappy. Most people who carry pain look outside themselves for help for a quick fix; for someone to love, listen to, or validate them; or numb their pain with food, alcohol or other substances. By not looking within and taking the time to hear our own body or even listen to what our soul is saying

---

[1] Glennon Doyle, *Love Warrior: A Memoir* (New York: Flatiron Books, 2016).

about the "you work" we need to do, we live in denial and become the victim of our circumstances.

We must cry, feel, and be brave to face our pain with vulnerability while expressing its energy by utilizing our talents. That's when we can call on our faith for support and kneel to heal. Our happy life and healing comes from facing our pain and aligning with our gifts and talents as if our life depends on it—because it does.

Exercise

When we feel physical pain, this meditation provides relief while not shying away from or avoiding what life is trying to teach us.

Pain Releasing Meditation:

Sit or lie down with your spine straight. Say a prayer to set your intention on releasing your pain, such as: "Dear God, please guide me in releasing the pain within and to surrendering it to you. Please surround and protect me with Your Divine love."

Begin cycle breathing, inhaling through your nose and exhaling out your mouth.

Bring your inhalation into your root chakra and hold the breath in your pelvic area to the count of ten.

As you release the breath, open your mouth and exhale outward with a deep sigh.

Repeat these steps three times, then sit and rest for a few minutes before continuing.

Now, bring the breath to an area of pain inside your body.

Hold the breath there to the count of ten, and very slowly exhale with control out your mouth.

Sit for several minutes.

Repeat if there are other areas of pain in the body.

Journal Prompts:

After completing the exercise, use the following prompts to write about your experience in your journal.

- What emotions came to the surface as you were doing this exercise?
- What sensations did you experience?

Healing Comes in Stages

Our healing doesn't just happen when we snap our fingers. What the Angels showed me long ago, when I began my own healing journey, is that our healing comes in layers, similar to those of an onion. If we peel one layer of the onion, another layer reveals itself, and the same is true of our healing. Just like that onion, when we begin to peel the layers apart and heal ourselves, we will start to tear up; deeper layers will make us cry and some layers will take our breath away. Healing our layers of pain opens space within our being for our gifts and talents to rise to the surface. Our willingness to participate in our healing and follow the twelve Goddess principles will certainly lead us to both understanding and confidently utilizing our gifts and talents.

What the Angels and the Divine have taught us here is that the twelve Goddess principles are meant for our soul's well-being. They're like a tune-up for our mind, body, and soul that guide us to release what no longer serves us and to welcome in positive new growth. When put into daily practice, they are the support system that keeps us functioning in high-vibrational, tip-top shape.

Connecting to the Divine

Our senses and chakras are connection points to God. When we align the energy that flows through these points with Source, our gifts open. Our faith is what supports the connection for the Divine to flow freely. Fear has the opposite effect: it is the stopping point for Divine energy. Our gifts can guide us as we move through various areas of our life. Faith in the guidance we receive through our gifts offers us an opportunity to let go of a preplanned outcome. That means we have to learn to let go of our need to control things; we have to stop plotting out the details of how our life will look. The subconscious triggers cause worry within us, which brings thoughts that arise and overshadow God's love for us. Without God's love, we don't feel safe and end up denying the guidance, mistrusting our gifts and turning off our connection. Our gifts are unique to us; no two souls will interpret the energy the same way. This is part of what makes you awesomely you!

As we connect to the Divine with our gifts, the energy flows through our senses and chakras. This is when the best part happens, just like the magic we believed in as a child. When we are in alignment with our Soul Self, we can clearly decipher the Divine energy. Then we become a Goddess with purpose!

The gifts that are connected to our chakras and senses are called the *clairs*. Most of us have one clair that is stronger than the others and becomes the most common way we connect. As we do our "you work," we may find that we also have several clairs onboard to support the dominant clair.

It can take a while for the dominant clair to reveal itself. I suggest that you take the time to meditate on the clairs with the following exercise to gain clarity. This will help you obtain a clear perspective for truth to flow in.

Exercise

This meditation is specifically designed to help you get in touch with your dominant clair or, if you are already in touch with it, with your supporting clairs.

Clairs Meditation:

Sit or lie down with your spine straight. Begin your cycle breathing, inhaling through your nose, exhaling out your mouth.

Allow your shoulders and hips to relax.

Bring your awareness inward as you follow your breath to meet with your root chakra at the base of your spine, holding it there for a few counts.

As you release your breath, follow the exhale upward.

On your next inhalation, bring your breath back to your root chakra and slowly bring your awareness up to your crown chakra.

With your next inhalation, feel yourself rising above your head so you are just above your body. Allow yourself to rise as high as you feel comfortable and visualize the following:

Just in front of your gaze is a white hallway. As you begin to walk down the hall, you notice a bright room to your right side. You step through the doorway into a beautiful room with white furnishings. There is a table with a vase of roses, pitcher of water, and a glass on it.

You walk over to the table and reach out to grasp the pitcher in your hand. You lift the pitcher and notice the water moving gently and begin to pour the water into the glass. When the glass is half-full, you place the pitcher back onto the table. You pick up the glass, feeling its coolness, and bring it up to meet your lips. Let yourself hear the water moving as you take a sip. You taste and feel the water as you swallow. You place the glass back down on the table and turn back toward the door.

As you walk back down the hall, you feel refreshed and happy.

Slowly you become aware of your body and your breathing. You start to feel connected to your muscles and can wiggle your fingers and toes.

When you are ready, open your eyes and move your body from side to side, becoming fully aware of your surroundings.

Journal Prompts:

After completing the exercise, use the following prompts to write about your experience in your journal.

- When you walked into the room, were you able see the table with the roses and the water pitcher?
- Were you able to smell the roses?
- Were you able to feel the pitcher or glass in your hand?

- Were you able to hear the water pouring from the pitcher into the glass or from the glass into your mouth?
- Could you taste the water?
- Could you feel the water inside your mouth as you swallowed?

Your answers can show you how you connect to energy through your senses. Take your answers and compare them to the clairs list on the following pages to get a better idea of which gifts you have opened.

The Seven Clairs and the Sensitive Soul

I shared this list of clairs in *The Goddess You*, and I think it's well worth repeating here! Following, you'll find a breakdown of the clairs, including their connection to the senses and their corresponding chakras. We can use this list to find our gift or gifts.

Don't fret; if you need more information, you can find details about the clairs at *believeangels.com*.

As you are reading, it is important to keep a few things in mind.

- While a clair will work with one main chakra, the clair will also heighten and work with all the chakras.
- The clairs, like chakras, can become off-balance and blocked, and therefore cause us to be hyposensitive instead of hypersensitive.
- The fact that we have a gift of connection doesn't necessarily mean that we are meant to pass messages to others.
- When opening our clairs, we can inadvertently invite fear energy into our being if we are not clear with our intention and connection to God.

1. ***Clairvoyance*** is the gift of clear seeing. People who are clairvoyant have a heightened sense of sight. This clair works mainly with the third eye and crown chakras. We may see Spirit or see colors and energy around others. When the gift of clairvoyance is off-balance, we will see shadow energy and may experience vivid dreams, including heightened dreams that inaccurately foretell future events. This is because psychic energy is the easiest energy to pick up, and

fear misleads us to believe in a destined outcome. Predictions and premonitions are often the work of fear energy.

2. ***Clairaudience*** is the gift of clear hearing. People who are clairaudient have a heightened sense of hearing. This clair works with our throat and third eye chakras. We can hear Spirit or energetic tones. When clairaudience is off-balance, we may be physically off-balance ourselves. We may also not be able to hear the truth. Hearing only negative fearful tones, as if everyone has it out for us, is the most common malfunction.

3. ***Clairsentience*** is the gift of clear feeling. People who are clairsentient have a heightened sense of feeling. This clair works with our throat and solar plexus chakras. We can feel Spirit or the energy of others around us. When the gift of clairsentience is off-balance, our feelings and pain level will be heightened, and we may experience severe digestive issues, aches throughout our body and dizziness. Being overly connected to emotions is a sign of malfunction.

4. ***Clairscent*** is the gift of clear smelling. People who have the gift of clairscent have a heightened sense of smell. This clair works with our throat chakra. We can smell Spirit or the energy surrounding us and others. When the gift of clairscent is off-balance, our sense of smell will be either closed or overly sensitive. We may also experience sinus, throat, and mouth disorders as the main malfunction.

5. ***Clairtangency*** is the gift of clear touch. People who have the gift of clairtangency have a heightened sense of touch. This clair works with our third eye and solar plexus chakras. We have the ability to connect with Spirit and energy through touch. When the gift of clear touch is off-balance, we will experience a heightened sensitivity to being touched. This can be experienced by us being drawn to touch others in ways they don't like, sometimes even to the point of abuse. It can also manifest with us not wanting to be touched.

6. ***Clairgustance*** is the gift of clear taste. People who have the gift of clairgustance have a heightened sense of taste. This clair works with our throat chakra. We have the ability to connect with and taste messages from Spirit or others. When the gift of clairgustance is off-balance, we will experience an acidic mouth and digestive system, causing certain foods to be bothersome. We can also be prone to mouth and tooth pain.

7. ***Clairempathy*** is the gift of clear knowing and emotion and a form of extrasensory perception. People who have the gift of clairempathy have a heightened sense of intuition, emotions, and feeling. This clair works with all our chakra points. We have the ability to connect to Spirit and others physically, emotionally, and intuitively almost as if they were within our body. When the gift of clairempathy is off-balance, we experience heightened and even unexplained feelings and emotions or uncontrollable mood swings, nightmares, and insomnia. We may also experience forms of depression and/or anxiety. It's important to note that while all people gifted with clairempathy are naturally empaths, an empath doesn't connect to Spirit in the same way that clairempaths can. It's not nearly as intense. The empath will experience emotions and symptoms or earth-bound energy, while the clairempath will have a nearly supernatural ability to connect with the emotions of others.

The Sensitive Soul is the most common gift of all. Though this is not a clair, I include it in this list as this gift is one that burdens most people because it is often misunderstood. It is less intense than being an empath and certainly less intense than clairempathy. The sensitive soul, also known as the *highly sensitive person*, feels energy on the outside of their body not inside. Our sense of feeling and emotions are heightened, and we can work with the heart and solar plexus chakras to develop this gift. This is very, very common in spiritually minded individuals—so much so that many mistakenly label themselves empaths when they are indeed not empaths.

When the gift of being a sensitive soul is off-balance, we may experience heightened empathy for others, issues around trying to control, being overly involved in other's lives or crying at the drop of a hat. We are more prone to get autoimmune diseases as the balance of this gift affects our central nervous system.

Karma, Energy, and Psychic Gifts

As with anything in life, whenever we take action, there is an opposite reaction that balances the energy, better known as *karma*. It is important for us to keep this in mind as we begin to work with our gifts.

Be forewarned, my friend, that if we choose not to do the "you work" of setting sacred space, praying and aligning with faith in God, we're inviting fear energy into our body. And that is no fun at all!

Interpreting energy comes easily for some and challenges others. Again, I will reiterate the importance of being in soul alignment here, because there are fear energies that lurk all around. And as you may recall from earlier in this book, fear is the easiest energy to pick up because it is an earth-bound energy. I've had hundreds of encounters with people who have had horrible experiences opening their gifts without being firmly aligned within God's graces. Many experienced visitations from darker or lower energies that turned their lives into a chaotic mess.

So as we can see, when we don't do the "you work" while aligning with God before opening our gifts, we can inadvertently pick up lower forms of energy. Trust me, nobody has time for that! Energy can be received and deciphered, as I shared with you earlier. And with that information in hand, I remind you that you now know about your receiving points: the senses and the chakras.

With that knowledge, let's dive further into understanding how psychic energy and Divine energy are received. Psychics connect to our life and the energy surrounding it on an earthly plane. They'll use this connection as a guide to deliver what they interpret and feel about our present situation and predict future events to come. Psychic energy can be one of the easiest energies to pick up and receive through our senses and chakras. This psychic energy is an earth-bound source and will also be interwoven with the energy of time, anger, resentment, judgment, past trauma, life events, and fear. An ethical psychic will weed out the fear tones and deliver a loving, insightful, and helpful reading. She or he will offer guidance that will aid us in moving forward with our lives. We should leave a reading with a positive outlook and with helpful and encouraging words that propel us forward in our life.

On the other hand, an unethical and low-vibrational psychic offers us a fear-based reading. While some of what they pick up on may have some truth to it, there is the absence of love energy, which means that the reading will leave us with worry and a definitive future outcome. Seeing the future this way has little to no merit for your life. This is for a couple of reasons: One, because the future of our soul is not written in stone, so while some things may be in our future, nothing is definite; and two, because of free will. God has provided us with free will, which means that although it might look like our life is going in one direction, we can choose to go in a completely different direction. Free will accounts for our choice to either go it alone or remember to choose God and love!

Mediums are psychics with an ability to connect to both earthly energy and to Heaven through what is known as the *veil*. The veil is also known as the bridge between Heaven and Earth. Since the veil is made of love, a person who is a medium is able to connect to the veil on many different levels, while also having areas of mediumship in which they specialize. A medium can specialize in the medical aspect of healing, like the medical medium, Anthony William; in validation of the departed, like the Long Island medium, Theresa Caputo; or in my case, spiritual alignment by facilitating healing for both physical and emotional pain. Mediums connect to Heaven through their special gifts and use their talents to deliver messages from the departed, Angels, as well as messages from God for our well-being.

As with some psychics, there are also some mediums who use their gift in an egotistical, fear-based way. Their type of readings leave us feeling fearful and anxious.

How can we know whether the person we're seeking out as a psychic or medium for a reading is of the highest caliber? We must simply ask our hearts if they are God-based and, of course, ask for references—just as we would for any other professional service.

Our Unshakable Faith

When our faith is unshakable, we can avoid picking up or getting stuck in pain and blocking the energy flowing through our senses and chakras. We no longer become paralyzed by doubt. We can take that leap of faith, make that life change, or take the time to nurture our soul with our talents.

Lessons are hard, my friend, there is no doubt about that. Yet every soul has to experience them. We are not alone in our resistance to change. The problem is that we isolate our fears and hold them close. We make excuses for why we can't change, for why we feel trapped, and for why our life seems so hard. Knowing how to work with our gifts and talents changes the old viewpoint and us along with it. No longer do we feel afraid to follow the guidance, make the changes that are best for us, and move forward with our life. We can stand with Divine love and bravely face our pain while expressing our talents and sharing our gifts with others!

CHAPTER EIGHT

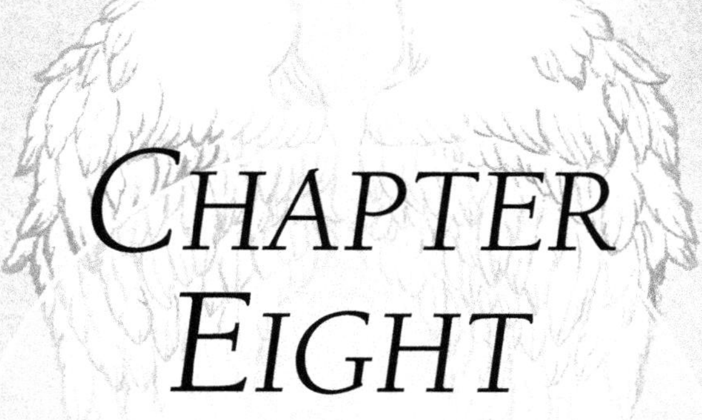

CHAPTER EIGHT

Pure of Heart

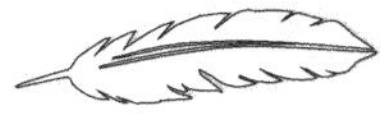

We are born with the gift of being our own healers through the connection to Spirit. We are born *pure of heart*. Our souls are energy sensitive and have come into life with the ability to channel Divine love and heal our deepest wounds. This pure love is woven through our DNA and energy centers. But the thing that makes a person who utilizes their gift of being a pure of heart different from those who don't, is that they move through life helping others. They become earth angels and their soul lesson and life path fuel them to feel and transmit love and light energy. They are like lighthouses, and the light they are meant to share with the souls they encounter throughout their life is that of Divine love. The pure of heart is a healer with a core soul connection to helping others.

A pure of heart person has an innocence about them that draws people in need to them. They connect to others pains easily and know why they feel what they feel. A pure of heart will connect to others and Divine energy and are usually empaths or sensitive souls. Of course, being energetically sensitive people, pure of hearts can become lost in the spiral of energy that surrounds them, because they absorb so much.

Pure of hearts are born into families of all walks of life. Family bloodlines will also pass down gifts and talents, such as certain clairs, artistic skills, and pure of hearts. Similar to DNA strands in bloodlines, these gifts that are passed down link Divine love and the voice of God through the generations. Of course, just like anyone else, these souls can become lost within their lives and lose the true source of who they are. The way home is to follow the twelve Goddess principles. By doing so, we can heal the separation from love.

We can know if we or a loved one is a pure of heart through a meditation and a series of questions that the Angels have shared. By opening our hearts, minds, and souls to God, we will begin to utilize our senses with our faith as a guide. This will lead us to the truth.

Keep in mind that the pure of heart soul will always have several clairs and always be either an empath or a sensitive soul. If you are unsure of your gifts, I invite you to return to and review the previous chapter.

Exercise

The purpose of this exercise is to connect you to your soul's truth so you can discover whether you or someone you love is a pure of heart.

Pure of Heart Meditation:

We start with a meditation. As with all meditations, get yourself into a comfy space to do this work. Be sure to grab your journal and pen!

Begin by setting your intention and saying the following prayer:

"Dear God, please surround me with Your Divine love and grace as I begin to align and understand the nature of [your or your loved one's name] soul's truth. I ask that You illuminate the truth while opening my heart. Amen."

Sit while practicing the cycle breathing for several minutes, allowing your body to rest, let go, and be still. Allow any thoughts to begin to dissipate as you release any tension you feel in your body with each exhale.

Bring your awareness, breath, and inner vision upward from the bottom of your feet to the top of your head. Invite each of your energy centers to open and flow with Divine love. As you reach the crown of your head, notice a burst of light as you lift ever so slightly upward. Your body is calm and still as your awareness moves higher and higher.

You're safe and loved as you find yourself standing in a Divine healing room. You are invited to witness the room filled with glistening white chairs and tables. As you look and walk about the room, you notice that one of the chairs has your name on it, inviting you to sit and rest. As you relax in your chair, you notice a notepad on the table beside you. You pick up the pen and instinctively feel that you should write down why you have come and what knowledge you are seeking. The words flow outward onto the glistening paper, and you feel relief rising inside your body.

Before you on the wall is a screen that begins to fill with writings. You adjust your eyes to make out the words and, as you do, without hesitation they become clear. You take time to read every word and feel the vibrations that they carry. You decide to write down in your journal each word being revealed. Be still and calm here as you record every word, emotion, and feeling that is being gifted in this moment.

When you have finished writing, bring your awareness back into your body, with your inner vision returning to the center of your forehead. Gently move your limbs as you notice the weight of your body return to this moment in time.

Take time to journal some more now that you are back on the physical plane. Notice the difference in your writing as you are now fully in your human form again.

Now that you have connected to the Divine and received your personal information, we can move on to explore the pure of heart questions. Take time to sit quietly and be in full alignment before you begin.

Quiz:

Consider the following questions, and then answer each one with a circle around the 'Y' for yes or 'N' for no:

1. ***The Spiritual Connection.*** Invite the presence of an Angel to come forward.

    - Can you physically see an Angel in front of you? Y or N
    - Can you see them in your mind? Y or N
    - Do you just know it is an Angel? Y or N
    - Are you able to hear them? Y or N
    - Can you reach out and feel the Angel? Y or N
    - Has God appeared to you? Y or N
    - Is this a symbolic form? Y or N
    - Is it a physical form? Y or N
    - Is it a knowing? Y or N

2. ***The Physical Connection.*** Think about what it is like to be around someone who is ill.

    - Can you describe the illness in detail? Y or N
    - Do you feel the illness in your body? Y or N
    - Do you know what it's like to take on another's personality? Y or N
    - Can you feel that person's energy inside your body? Y or N
    - Can you feel that person's emotional state of being? Y or N
    - Do you cry when others cry? Y or N
    - Do you feel others' sadness? Y or N
    - Can you feel the emotions of someone even when you're communicating electronically? Y or N

3. ***The Mental Connection.*** Think of what it feels like when someone is angry with you.

- Do you feel separated from love? Y or N
- Do you feel separated from that person? Y or N
- Can you feel the chatter of another person's thoughts? Y or N
- When someone is working next to you, do you know what they are doing without physically looking at them? Y or N
- Do you learn by reading? Y or N
- Do you learn by doing? Y or N
- Do you have prophetic dreams? Y or N
- When someone is talking about you, do you know? Y or N
- Do you feel that energy in your body? Y or N
- Have you thought about or felt something that later came true? Y or N

Now count the answers to tell the bigger story. You may have already noticed a pattern but take a moment to look over the answers again and then complete the following chart.

Sections:	Total Yes Answers:
1. The Spiritual Connection:	
2. The Physical Connection:	
3. The Mental Connection:	
Grand Total Yes Answers:	

Quiz summary:

Pure of Heart: 24–27 yes answers
Empath: 14–23 yes answers
Sensitive Soul: 1–13 yes answers

Knowing Our Path

Not knowing if we are an empath, a sensitive soul, and/or have come here as a pure of heart to channel Divine love, will increase our inner turmoil. The daughter of my client, Judy, offers an example of how lost someone can become when they don't understand that they are picking up energy from others or why they feel the way they feel. The unfortunate epidemic of our society is that we do not talk openly about or teach our children about energy or connecting to Divine Source. As a society, we separate from the truth of our equality and energetic connection to all living things.

Judy was in great sorrow. I knew as soon as she booked her reading that it was going to be very emotional. I could feel her grief before she entered my office. I sat, as I always do, with my legs crossed in my corner chair. Judy was sitting on the sofa and appeared stoic. But I felt her energy and saw her truth; I knew her suffering as my own. My body shivered, my spine, though straight, was weakened, and my knees were numb. I silently told the Angels, *I don't know how this woman walked in here on her own.* In reply, I was impressed with the message of a suicide. We began with my introduction on how I work with Spirit and how the work I do as a medium is always connected to healing. As soon as I put pen to paper, her daughter stepped forward. I put the pen down and looked at Judy as I spoke. My voice shook as I repeated her daughter's words, "I'm so sorry, Mama, it's not your fault." Her daughter then asked me to sit next to her mom and hug her to show her emotion and connect with her mom even more. I shared with Judy what her daughter was asking of me, and Judy consented to receive a hug. We sat in an embrace as she let go, melting into my shoulder, crying. I could feel her daughter sitting right there with us the whole time, as if she were a part of me.

When we sat back, I looked into Judy's eyes and shared what had happened. Her daughter said she was an empath and had lived in a constant turmoil of feelings and emotions that she did not understand. She covered the chaos she felt within her mind and her body with several forms of addictions. She became more and more confused from the energy she was feeling in her body as time went by and could no longer find the calm she longed for. She took responsibility for taking her life, ending it with an overdose while numbing the energy in her being that made no sense to her.

Judy sobbed as she confirmed that her daughter struggled her entire life with heightened emotions. Her daughter also spoke of her mother shutting herself off from the world since she died, saying her mom was normally very social and loved the holidays. Judy confirmed this, saying she hadn't been able to face others or put up her holiday decorations she normally loved so much. Her daughter spoke of an upcoming family dinner that was in the planning stage, where her mother had invited her birth father to join Judy and her husband. Her daughter showed me a photograph being put into a frame and being shared as a remembrance. She asked her mother to do this with love rather than sorrow. Judy was awestruck as she had just made copies of her favorite photo of her daughter and planned to give it as a gift to her daughter's father.

Judy shared how loving her daughter was to others, always lending a hand or being there when someone was in need. Yet she watched her daughter plummet while trying everything she knew to help her get well. Therapy in facility treatment centers were not enough for this lovely young woman who was plagued with the emotions and pains of others.

The reading brought release and relief to Judy, along with the knowing that her daughter was safe and still with her.

Life as an Empath

Living as an empath can be challenging and depleting. *The Empath's Survival Guide*, by Judith Orloff, is an excellent resource that I have recommended to clients and students who suffer from the harsh side effects of their empathic abilities. It even goes into the details of the science about empathy and what happens in the brain. Dr. Orloff writes:

> Empaths have an extremely reactive neurological system. We don't have the same filters that other people do to block out stimulation. As a consequence, we absorb into our own bodies both the positive and stressful energies around us. We are so sensitive that it's like

> holding something in a hand that has fifty fingers instead of five. We are truly "super responders."
>
> Research shows that high sensitivity affects approximately 20 percent of the population, though the degree of one's sensitivity can vary. Empaths have often been labeled as "overly sensitive" and told to "get a thicker skin." As children and adults, we are shamed for our sensitivities rather than supported. We may experience chronic exhaustion and want to retreat from the world because it often feels so overwhelming.[2]

More often than not, when I meet with a client who is depressed, I am shown the signs of that person being an empath. Depression is very real, and the causes can stem from genetics to life experiences to pure karma. As a healer, the Angels show and impress upon me where each client's depression originates. I see genetic or chemical imbalance as a lulled energy flow in the brain. When it is depression, I see the word *depression* in writing in front of me and feel the client's despair in my body.

When someone is an empath and doesn't know it, I feel a tornado of emotions welling through my body that make me feel dizzy and tired. When a person knows they are an empath and uses their energy to control, manipulate, or hurt others, I feel as if an anger is rising from within and an energetic righteousness washes over my being. There are many aspects to a person who is an empath. Once an empath comes to terms with their gifts and how they can use them, they can utilize their energy for good, for clear intuitive guidance, and/or for helping others. An empath who is moving and grooving in their energy in a healthy state will be uplifted when working with others. They will still experience the energy around them but will do so without taking it on as part of their being. A healthy empath is able to decipher the different layers and tones of energy as they channel Divine love to the other person.

---

[2] Judith Orloff MD, *The Empath's Survival Guide: Life Strategies for Sensitive People* (Louisville: Sounds True, 2017).

Now we can move forward with a new understanding of what it means to live as an energetically sensitive person. The empath who is affected by earth-bound energy can feel and take on other beings' energy within their bodies. A sensitive soul who feels the earth-bound energy on the outside of their body is equally challenged by it. And the pure of heart, who can be either an empath or a sensitive soul, has an extrasensory ability to connect to Spirit and channel Divine love; in fact, they have a mission.

We are all here for a reason. Each of us is on a journey to find our own personal meaning in life, including our purpose for being here, but this will only come to us when we practice the "you work" to know more about ourselves.

Chapter Nine

CHAPTER NINE

What God Wants Us to Know

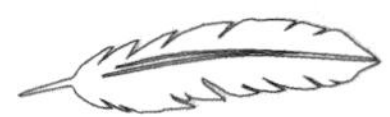

"Don't let your hearts be troubled. Trust in God, and trust also in me."
—JOHN 14:1 NLT

Love is always available to us. Whether we are going through a divorce, facing an illness, facing bankruptcy, or grieving the loss of a loved one, we crave love. We feel separated, discouraged, even angry that we are alone to face these things before us. We wonder why we can't feel God or His love. He seems nowhere to be found during our lowest of lows. But here's the good news: God has a few things He wants you to know.

What God Wants You to Know

Here are the top three things Divine Source would have you remember:

1. ***He loves you.*** We are the spark of love. His love lives within us. Our strength is always bigger than we believe.

2. ***You are invaluable.*** We are all meant to be here, and you are perfect in his eyes!

3. ***Forgiveness sets you free.*** We have been given this most awesome gift, a chance to be our best self and to set free those who have caused us pain.

Let's recap some of the important details from the previous chapters:

- Divine energy is received through our energy centers, also known as our chakras.
- Energy is deciphered through our senses.
- Our intention and faith are the foundation that keep our mind, body and soul in balance.
- Knowing Shmego's tone is key to living in our soul alignment.
- The present moment is our happy spot.
- Psychic energy is the easiest energy to pick up on.
- Free will is a gift from God that gives us the opportunity to choose love in each moment.
- Everyone has a past and lessons to work through; no one is above or below us.

Of course, there are always the finer details of what God wants you to know. First, raising our energy to meet the Divine is how we can connect with ease. This is how mediums channel our loved ones and angelic messages. Remember, though: it is not about telling the future. That is not what God wants for us. Rather, healing messages are meant to support our journey and heal stagnant energy. This is how the messages, guidance, and connections to our departed loved ones are intended to be used. They offer gentle guidance from above with the infusion of love!

Connecting our chakras to God and Divine love will ensure that we don't pick up any lower psychic energy. This is because God wants us to have the best life experience possible. In order for us to live our best life, it's über important that we begin by choosing to do so, and then commit ourselves to do the "you work." Nothing comes easily, yet when we do the "you work" to shift our perceptions and heal, we are relieved of the trapped energy. That's when ease sets in.

God speaks to all life. We can turn on our receptors by opening our senses and our chakras to hear Him. Most people only turn to God when they experience great pain or fear, but God wants to hang out with us every day! Having a relationship with heavenly beings will improve our mood, lift our view of the world, and keep us focused on the present moment. God says that we are perfectly imperfect, and he forgives us for everything.

In fact, there is absolutely nothing we can do that will not be forgiven. This is a hard thing for most humans to believe, because of the human history of violence that has been a part of the planet for centuries. Even with the devastation of war and violence that appears throughout time, reminding us that evil exists, God says love is still available. The people who hurt others and devalue human life are God's children, meaning: Yes, He loves them as He loves you. How is it that God can love evil? God is the Father, and like any parent, His children do wrong things. God is not happy about that, nor does He condone what has been done against Him, but He will discipline with love and forgiveness because that is the role of a good parent.

Judgment

Will people be punished for the evil they unleash on another? God says that punishment and soul judgment is something all His children experience during the purification stage. This happens through teaching the soul about the pain that it caused. No act of hate is forgiven without the soul first going through purification.

There are ancient teachings dating back before Jesus Christ that present purgatory as a continuous state wherein the soul is left to suffer in a state of everlasting purification. Purgatory, as the Angels have shown me, is the holding point for the soul, where the soul is given the choice to be freed from the evil with which it has been poisoned during the life cycle. This decontamination of fear energy takes time, and again, time in the afterlife does not exist as it does here, so it is not measurable. During this stage, the soul is in this state of being still, but love is fully available to the soul as soon as it chooses love over fear.

Because this is a process made of love, not of hate, there is no separation from Divine love unless the soul so chooses. The soul can separate from love, from God, and choose eternal damnation. This is known as falling from grace. A soul will choose to do this if fear is the prevalent force of evil and has overcome the soul. But remember that at any time, the soul can choose love by asking for forgiveness!

How Fear Manipulates

Fear is sneaky, as we have learned. With that truth now revealed, learning the ways that fear manipulates our thoughts in everyday life can illuminate the process of how fear morphs its energy into evil.

Let's break this down step-by-step so we can have a clear understanding of how the process of fear can take over a life.

1. ***Separation from love.*** This happens for most during childhood, from the conditioning and belief systems of the adults in our life. This conditioning might teach us that we aren't smart, that we behave badly, are mean, are funny-looking, or have big ears.

2. ***Living in the past.*** This is when we are unable to let go of the first separation from love, and the past feelings and emotions hold us in a victim state.

3. ***Denial of love.*** This is when we have little to no faith and are living disconnected from the Divine.

Jesus teaches that sharing the phases of fear will illuminate where we may be stuck in our thoughts, actions or reactions. It's also an opportunity for us to witness others with a compassionate heart—for where we infuse love into a thought, feeling or emotion of another, we also heal a layer of fear within ourselves.

Life's path brings us love at all crossroads. Our soul's journey will bring us toward difficulty in order to teach us that we will have to examine and practice our faith. *God's will be done.* This truthful prayer is what we need to remember as we navigate through life. But we often worry and stress about our preferred outcome instead of focusing on love and trusting God. When we do this, we end up forcing our desires as the best outcome. All because we forget that faith has our back. Furthermore, we're unable to see that God's will for us is far more healing than our desires, which are often laced with fear's energy and set up by Shmego himself.

The cool thing is that now that we know Shmego is indeed the enemy, he will leave us feeling like the lyrics from an old country and western song where we lose our wife, our life, our job, and so on. Play the record backward and you get your spouse and life back, your job is better, and everything becomes rosy again. Life is an experience to be enjoyed. God wants that for you; he wants us to choose love and be proud of our choice to align with love. God also says it is better to be inspired, to lead with love than it is to lead without love.

Letting go of control is not in most people's nature. "Success" is often a misinterpreted mission that causes a separation from the will of the Divine. Many strive to build a career without full awareness of how their life path and authentic truths are to be used as a service to others, seeing life as a competitive race instead. Manipulating an outcome rather than manifesting with God is how some choose to meet their wants and desires. This form of life is never one of service but one that serves the "I," and it comes with a price. Yes, they will seem to have money and even happiness, but what we don't see is the karmic energy that builds over time or the fact that the things they acquire along the way actually deplete their energy. The end result is unhappiness and feeling unfulfilled, because the more we get the more we want, and it seems like our cup is never full.

Most of us can relate to this on some level. I know I can! In *The Goddess You*, I shared a story about the shoe boutique I used to own, Sassy Shoe. Back then, I wanted so badly to be successful. I also felt the need to prove myself to others, and I did this by trying to impress my family and friends with my new business. I gave everyone I knew a special discount. I worked really hard for my desired outcomes. I prayed and prayed for success. At one point, I even had a sweet friend who offered to pray a *novena*, a special prayer that is said for nine consecutive days, for my little boutique.

Instead of following my original business plan and intuition, I extended both my generosity and my finances too far. I knew the second I made the decision to purchase more inventory than I could afford that I was going against my truth. Yet the voice within, that Shmego guy, told me that my boutique deserved more product, that I was foolish not to buy more to make others happy and that by extending the line of credit, I was showing others that I was a smart business owner. None of that was true. I made the choice to go it alone. I didn't pray on it or ask for help from anyone I admired. I just wanted to be successful, and I would do what I had to do to prove it.

As time went by, I was shown that my desire to prove myself had a reverse effect. I stopped purchasing what the business could not afford and no longer gave everyone I knew a discount, but by then it was too late to save the business.

Despite closing my business, I don't look at the time I spent at Sassy Shoe as a loss in general. Rather, I look back on my little boutique fondly. It taught me many valuable lessons not just about business but about myself too. I understand now that God wants us to have success. Partnering with Him and using the resources He provides me with keeps me on my path and spiritually aligned. Now, God is my business partner and I always feel supported.

Exercise

The lovely novena that follows brings us back into our heart center and connects us with the God-spark within us. It is a prayer that is meant to be practiced for nine consecutive days and includes an exercise for releasing energy. This can help us let go of any of the following: judgment, anger, pain, trauma, confusion, depression, anxiety or blocks. On the positive end, it can also help us open space within to welcome abundance. We can also use this novena when we are working on accomplishing a goal, when we are facing a challenge, when we need courage or when we are lost in our life. This is a beautiful and intentional prayer that will amplify the love in your life!

How to prepare for saying the novena:

- Plan ahead, as it's ideal to say the novena the same time each day during the nine consecutive days.
- Set an altar with items that inspire you, such as religious items, crystals, or candles.
- Keep a dedicated journal and pen by the altar.
- On day one, before you start, write down the intention for your novena in your journal or on a piece of paper that can be put on the altar.

This novena is meant to open our hearts to our Soul Self by releasing energy that no longer serves us. Repeat the novena for three consecutive days and on the third day, do the release exercise. Then repeat the entire process two more times.

Align and Release Novena:

Novena (days 1–9)

Read your intention and sit with your hands on your heart for a few moments with reverence for yourself.

Sit with your spine straight and feet planted on the floor. Place your hands on your lap with palms facing upward and close your eyes. Allow your tongue to relax off the roof of your mouth and your shoulders to release tension and drop down.

Begin with several rounds of the cycle breathing, inhaling in through the nose, exhaling out of the mouth. Feel your body release tension as your inner gaze focuses on your heart center.

With the next nine inhalations repeat these words, either mentally or out loud: I am that I am. With every exhalation, repeat: I am the grace of God.

After you have repeated the novena nine times, place your hands palm over palm on your heart center. Inhale, filling your chest cavity with air, and hold it to the count of nine.

Slowly exhale the breath as you lift your shoulders up toward your ears and hold them there for a few seconds. Then bring your shoulders toward your back, lowering them down and pressing out your "wings" while pushing your heart forward, repeating three more times: I am that I am. I am the grace of God. Release your arms downward.

Stay here until you are ready to gently move your body side to side, roll your shoulders, wiggle your fingers and toes, and slowly open your eyes.

Journal—Novena:

Write in your journal about how you are feeling and any experiences you had.

Release Exercise (days 3, 6, and 9)

Following the novena, place your hands palm over palm on your heart center. Then repeat the following steps three times:

Step 1: Inhale your breath to the area within your body in which you feel physical pain or anywhere you may be holding energy that no longer serves you. Hold the breath in this space for a count of ten.

Step 2: Slowly exhale the breath outward, adding a sigh at the end of the exhalation.

Step 3: Again, slowly exhale the breath as you lift your shoulders up toward your ears and hold them there for a few seconds. Then bring your shoulders toward your back, lowering them down and pressing out your "wings" while pushing your heart forward, repeating three more times: I am that I am. I am the grace of God. Release your arms downward.

Stay here until you are ready to gently move your body side to side, roll your shoulders, wiggle your fingers and toes, and slowly open your eyes.

Journal—Release Exercise:

Write in your journal about how you are feeling and any experiences you had.

Our Inner Being

We will experience a renewal of our energy each time we choose to focus on our inner world rather than try to control our outer world. When we release our hold over outcomes and agendas we soften within, allowing for the spark of Divine love to guide us.

Every time we practice a meditation, say a prayer or sit in stillness, we are participating in our spiritual wellness. The time we reflect within, doing our "you work," will reinforce our efforts with personalized revelations that restore our mind, body, and soul. God wants this for each of us.

When we say "Amen" at the end of a prayer or mantra, it means we agree with the statement, and so it is. This aligns us with Divine truth and intention.

The three life-changing takeaways from this moment are: You are loved unconditionally. Amen. You are invaluable. Amen. Forgiveness will always free and heal you. Amen.

CHAPTER TEN

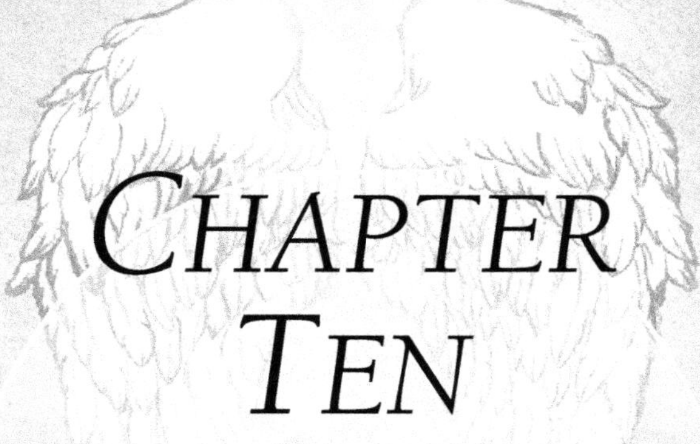

CHAPTER TEN

How Love Can Support Us

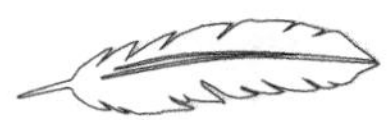

"God loves each of us as if there were only one of us."

— *SAINT AUGUSTINE*

Love is pure. When influenced by logic and fear, the human mind cannot grasp the entire meaning of love. Love, as described by Wikipedia, is "a variety of different feelings, states, and attitudes that range from interpersonal affection to pleasure." Love is also described as an emotion, a virtue and an action, meaning it's a choice, not a feeling. Feelings come and go, rise and fall. Love remains.

Love is so vast in energy that it is not easily confined by the walls of the mind. Like religions that teach within four walls and contain us under an umbrella of their belief system, we also have walls around our personal beliefs about love and God. The vastness of love and God is within us. We are the foundational dwelling in which God, spirituality, love, compassion, faith, joy, and hope all reside. And just like with religion, there is no right or wrong way to worship; rather, there is just room for expansion in our personal relationship with love and God. Think of it as having a skylight open during a religious service. There is far greater love available when we open our personal skylight, which is our crown chakra.

Let's go on a little journey to experience what this means for us. Go ahead and grab your journal and find a comfortable place to do the dream palace exercise.

Exercise

This exercise will help open your crown chakra to let love in.

Dream Palace:

Start by setting the intention that you be surrounded by Divine love.

Say the following prayer of petition: "Dear Lord, guide me as I open my crown chakra. I invite Your love to shine within me, opening new areas of my body, mind, and soul to love while allowing me to witness the wisdom of truth rushing through me. Amen."

Take time to do several rounds of cycle breathing—in through the nose, out through the mouth.

As you begin to settle into your calm, I invite you to begin to imagine your very own dream palace. This is the most beautiful home you can imagine, set in the precise center of the most spectacular walled garden, with every detail created to your exact specification.

Visualize your palace. Nothing but fear can stop you from dreaming of your beautiful space, so at this point take a moment to set another loving intention. Consciously decide to keep fear from penetrating the outside walls of your palace.

Breathe in and be still for a moment.

Keeping your eyes closed, take time to envision your entire palace. Imagine walking the land within your palace walls. Notice the layout of the land, smell the fragrances in the air, feel the warmth of the earth under your feet as you walk through your gardens. Notice what the exterior of the building in the center looks like.

Now start to walk toward the entrance of your palace. As you walk through the front door of your dream palace, become aware of all that is there to see, use all your senses to explain the comfort of your palace. Your knowing tells you that your palace is your safe place to be your Soul Self.

As you walk around the main level, notice the many windows, doors, and hallways. Recall the outside of your palace and notice that the inside has seemingly endless space with many staircases and passageways for you to discover. The palace has the feeling of being familiar yet also of being foreign.

You decide to follow one particular passageway that leads you through a cool and darker area. You notice that you feel safe but uneasy because of the unknown. Then you recall that fear does not dwell within the palace walls, so you call on love to lead the way. Love immediately illuminates the passageway as your faith rises to the surface.

The coolness of this space tells you a story, a tale of a heart that is opening on a new level. You find your way to a beautiful room filled with your favorite flowers. The scent is heavenly, as are the furnishings. You decide to sit in this room and enjoy the surroundings and the newfound energy. As you are resting within this sacred space, your body is flooded with sensations of love. The room fills with love's energy as you witness this miracle moment. Your senses are wide open, and your body begins to absorb the many levels of love available at this moment.

Stay in this room, taking time to write freely in your journal while your senses are heightened. Write down your feelings and emotions of being in love. Be still as long as you need before bringing your awareness to your breathing. Take several deep breaths as you become aware of the here and now, bringing your attention to the room you are in. Move your fingers, toes, and neck. One more deep breath and you are back in this moment.

The palace gardens represent our soul and its expansiveness, while the palace within them represents our physical body. Being one with our Soul Self allows us to experience love on many levels.

This beautiful exercise can be repeated over and over. Each time reveals another room, hall, passageway, staircase, or window to experience. Every time we visit our palace, we open to more love.

We are that palace and home which we built in our imagination. The many gardens we witnessed are Heaven's promises to us. The unending rooms, windows, hallways, and passageways are the spaces where God wants to be with us. When we close off a doorway to love, such as from trauma or grief, and don't allow ourselves to witness the lessons the experience has to offer us, we are shutting off the flow of love.

Journal Prompts:

After completing the exercise, use the following prompts to write about your experience in your journal.

- Think of a time when you were forcing an outcome and write it down.
- How did you feel about yourself during that time?
- What lessons can you see now that you have a new perspective?

Love Has Our Back

Love will direct us to experience the expansiveness of its energy. Love supports us—if we allow it to! Remember, love is not simply defined because the human mind needs logic, so we force words to define meanings, things, and even experiences in order to make sense out of them. Love cannot be defined as just one word, feeling, or thing because love will not satisfy the human mind by being blocked in; it is against the nature of God to do so.

Expansive thinking leads us to our soul's wisdom. Wisdom is God's gift to all humanity. Each soul can tap into higher consciousness if they choose to do so. We can choose the path toward the Soul Self to connect to our higher wisdom and dwell in love.

Joanie's story demonstrates this.

She felt unworthy of living when she came for a reading. As we began, I could immediately feel the pain she was carrying in her body. Some of her pain felt like it was coming from grief, which appears as a heaviness in my chest, and then I was led by Spirit to feel her nerve endings sparking in a constant flare. Her brother stepped forward first, claiming Joanie as his sister. He impressed a sharp pain in the back of my head as a sign of how he departed, along with an unplugged, flying feeling that indicated a quick departure.

Joanie confirmed that her brother had fallen off his bike when he was five years old, hitting his head and becoming unconscious. Joanie and her friend dragged her brother into the house while screaming for help. Her mother called the ambulance, but by the time the paramedics arrived, he was barely breathing. He later passed away at the hospital. Her brother impressed into my body the great grief that his sister had been carrying, and her sorrow reflected back to me as a depression she was trapped in.

Joanie had spent her whole life not trusting the men in her life as she lived with a constant fear they would leave her. This, along with her feeling that she was not worthy of living, could only be healed when she addressed and processed the grief from her brother's tragic death.

When grief is trapped within the body and unhealed, it has a negative effect on a person's well-being. In Joanie's case, she lived with constant physical pain after a lung cancer surgery. The pain nagged at her through sparking nerve endings in her back and chest wall. Not only that, but these constant sensations also kept her feeling stranded, isolated, and alone—exactly the way she'd felt when her brother died. Joanie was desperate for relief and had been thinking of taking her own life.

We spoke about how her brother's soul was only meant to live those few short years and that his dying was part of a greater collective lesson for both Joanie and her mother. Her brother then impressed the guilt that their mother still endured daily from the choices she made all those years ago. She had often wondered whether driving the boy to the hospital instead of waiting for the ambulance may have saved his life. He impressed an image of his hand on his mother's shoulder, standing next to her as a man rather than the boy she remembered. Joanie burst into tears as she felt her mother's grief. As he stood next to his mother, his words were loving and filled with healing energy. Joanie received these words and this energy and promised to relay them to her mother. It was a healing that they had both been longing for.

The Angels guided me to share some pain management tips for Joanie that would help ease the suffering behind her physical pain. I also shared with her another fact that the Angels have illuminated to me over time: our pain is a reminder of something gone wrong. For true healing to take place, we need to find the layers that brought us to the point of that pain and heal them, one layer at a time. For most things, there isn't a quick fix; rather, there's a slow, meaningful healing where love supports our efforts to face what we need to face. By sharing a short but effective meditation with Joanie, I helped her rewitness her childhood and detach from the pain to see where love had been available to her, even at the moment of her brother's death and along the hard road that followed.

The vastness of our soul awakens us as we heal our past perceptions. It's important to remember that love has our back as we venture to these new uncharted places within our being. Loving another is easy, but loving ourselves is not always so easy. Finding our reflection of our truest self, our Soul Self, will remind us of our worthiness. We are meant to be here to experience love and to remember how this mystical gift supports us on every level.

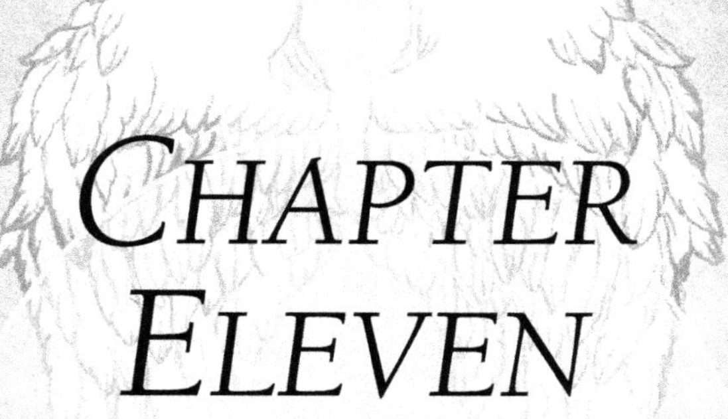

Chapter Eleven

CHAPTER ELEVEN

SAINTS AND SINNERS

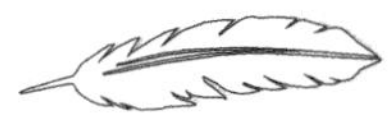

"Hate the sin, love the sinner."

— *MAHATMA GANDHI*

Saints are souls that have lived with the promise that love offers them, as well as to those they serve. They have been guided to serve humanity through various charitable actions. A saint is known as someone who was embodied to live in a state of holiness and to dedicate their life to Divine law.

Sinners are also souls that live and have lived with the fear of love's promises. They are living beings who have committed an act that is against Divine law and God.

Sinners, like saints, share the same calling and guidance to serve humanity. Unlike saints, who serve God and Divine law, sinners serve others with the intention of gaining from their service.

You may be wondering why this makes them a sinner. It is not the desire to have an equal exchange for a service that makes one a sinner. No, that's not it at all. Rather, a sin is when the heart is attached to an outcome instead of being dedicated to service and to faith. This goes against God and Divine law. So while we may have sinned, we can always choose to change our life path and walk as a saint does. Devoting one's life to serving God is compassion at its finest.

Turning a life from one of a sinner to one of a saint is not out of reach. We spoke earlier about forgiveness and healing fear, and it is through these actions that we can shift our thoughts and be of service.

The Truth about Manifesting

The practice of manifesting has gained attention over the past few years. As the internet has increased the availability of information, many people are now teaching the age-old knowledge of how easy it is to get what we desire. And it works! But the truth is that the action of manifesting can easily become a sinful act.

As discussed earlier in this book, our desires are the things we wish to come to us. Those desires may or may not be in our highest interest; they may or may not be in alignment with our Goddess truths. Manifesting without first connecting to God can actually set us up for a huge crash. Sure, we may receive all those desires we have longed for; we may even use this power for altruism, sharing our wealth with others, but we will miss our soul's chance to experience valuable and timely lessons that are needed for our soul's well-being. The big truth is that our lessons are the very reason we are here in the first place; our souls are here to experience them in this lifetime. Going it without God is both irresponsible and dangerous.

Jack's story illustrates this.

He and his wife booked a reading together. They were struggling in many ways from the harsh life they had been living since Jack had lost his job a few years earlier. As they entered my office, I could feel the lull in energy from both of them. The Angels illuminated the separation from Jack's Soul Self and said that, while he believed in God, he was not allowing love into his being. I could also see the soulmate connection between them, but the love-energy light was dulled. The Angels immediately impressed a metal taste in my mouth, which is my sign for medication. Jack confirmed that he was taking both an antidepressant as well as an antianxiety medication.

Jack's father stepped forward, embracing his son with a warm, heavenly hug. He then proceeded to hang his head low, which is my sign of a soul sharing an apology. He spoke of how hard he was on his son and admitted that he had abused his son both physically and emotionally. As tears streamed down Jack's face, I continued to channel his father's words. The father shared that Jack worked very hard to support his family at a job that did not serve his soul. He also shared that Jack was a sensitive soul who was being bullied by others in the workplace. Jack wanted to dismiss some of what his father was saying, because he lived with the deep-seated pain of his father's abuse, but I could see that he knew every word his father said was true.

Remember, the act of departing this world involves a massive purification. No matter how difficult a person may have been in life, in death they are much more evolved. It can be hard to remember this especially when we've been hurt by someone who claimed to love us. Jack's father's act of coming forward and taking responsibility for his actions with love brought an incredible healing. This is a reflection of how one who has sinned can heal both their soul and free another. Eventually, Jack accepted what his father had to say and became visibly lighter.

As we continued, Jack remembered how a former coworker would manipulate and berate him about his work. Jack's life lesson was around using his voice to speak up, and this was becoming illuminated through the painful relationships in his life. When Jack was laid off he took it to heart, thinking he was at fault. Jack's father shared that the man who bullied Jack was a jealous man. He revealed that this man had lied to Jack's boss, resulting in Jack losing his job. Hearing the news that his coworker had lied was another level of healing Jack needed. His father then explained how, though his coworker had sinned, it had actually helped Jack on his path by exposing his life lesson and bringing him closer to his PMC.

Jack's father shared all this for a reason: Jack needed to see how love was available to him and how he was not a victim. His obsession to find new work was taking a toll on his relationship. His wife felt him sinking further into depression with every failed lead. Jack was forcing his agenda with God through praying for what he thought was best for him and his family. Jack's father then spoke about his son's gifts and passions and how he could better serve his family and others by sharing his talents. He urged his son to begin writing. He showed me that Jack could use his voice and love of God to help guide others who suffered the effects of bullying in the workplace. Jack said he loved to write and had once thought of being a writer. As he spoke this aloud and shared these childhood memories, his whole body lit up.

The actions taken by both Jack's father and coworker were sinful. Yet Jack needed to forgive them for his own healing to take place. He needed to see his life lesson and step into his true mission on the planet. The Angels shared that the act of forgiveness would set Jack free from the pains of the past and that self-love would carry Jack forward to manifest abundance and to live with love.

Manifesting with God always provides us with truthful insights. It brings clarity to the Divine timing at play. In return for the "you work" we do as we manifest, we heal and grow while we experience joy. By participating as the saint of our own life, we actually get to be of service, heal, and receive. Sainthood therefore is not out of our reach. This doesn't mean that everyone is meant to become a religious saint; in fact, that sort of sainthood is quite rare. Yet a life of being in service, of walking within our soul's truth, is filled with moments that call us to serve with faith as our guidepost and receive what we're meant to receive in Divine time.

Exercise

This exercise will help us manifest with God. The first time you do this meditation it can be more general, but after that, you can set your intention to connect with a specific area of your life. As you put this meditation into practice regularly, you will find that manifesting is about finding ease as you move through your life's challenges and live your soul's truths.

Manifest with God:

Begin with setting your intention to connect to God.

Say the following prayer of protection: "Dear God, please surround me and fill me with Your Divine love. I ask that your love shield me from any fears that arise and that my soul's truths are illuminated brightly. Amen."

Sit in a meditative position with your spine straight and your palms open and resting on your legs. Start the cycle breath as you settle yourself into the here and now.

Allow your body to absorb the oxygen that comes in with each deep inhalation. Feel your muscles let go with every exhale.

With your eyes closed, focus on your third eye chakra. Allow any thoughts to simply pass by as you remain present in this moment.

Using your right middle finger, gently begin tapping slowly on your heart center. As the breath enters, it gently flows inward, connecting and igniting love energy to flow.

Move your hand to your third eye chakra and gently begin tapping slowly on the center of your forehead.

With your next inhalation, invite the breath and love to flow in through your third eye.

Just be present as you automatically take another inhalation through your third eye. Notice the heart chakra begin to engage with the energy from the third eye, swirls of energy interlocking and expanding.

Bring your hand now to your crown chakra and begin slowly tapping as your internal eyesight focuses on the crown. With your intention, invite the flow of love energy to the crown chakra.

Relax your hand and place it back on your lap.

As your crown begins to open, a rush of energy connects to the flow that already connects your third eye and heart chakras. The three chakras are expanding with the purest form of Divine light energy.

Feel yourself begin to float and lift your view until you are just above your physical body. Notice that here within this energy is the connection to your Soul Self. Merge with this Divine energy, feeling at peace and surrounded by God's love. Your awareness begins to flow upward as if you were in a spiritual elevator. As you rise your body feels safe, your mind is filled with calm, and the excitement of love's promises fills you with peace.

Stay here in this celestial place for a few breaths, and then step forward into what can only be described as a cloud. Notice a beautiful chair in front of you and sit down. Feel the presence of the Angels inviting you to be safe and loved. The movement of air, the gentleness of the light, and the soft musical sounds comfort you.

It is now that the Angels bring forth your higher self, who comes to float in front of you. As your eyes focus on the figure before you, your heart fills with gratitude, noticing all the beauty of your Soul Self. Take time to be still with this moment.

Now that you are surrounded by Angels and God's love, you can connect with your soul's truth. You are able to speak or think a question or desire and immediately receive confirmation. You are filled with hope as your answers gently flow through your being. Allow the energy to bring peace to the points you struggle with.

When the time to return comes, it is natural and calm. The Angels gently guide you back to your physical body. You feel your energy heightened as you enter this moment in time with ease. Your awareness is back in your body. Your heart is full, and your mind is calm. Move first your fingers, then your arms, and then your feet before opening your eyes.

Journal:

Write in your journal about how you are feeling and any experiences you had.

Releasing Sin

While we all may sin, we don't have to live life as sinners. The truth is that we can heal and grow from the experience of sinning if and when we fully admit that we have sinned. They say that the two hardest things to do in life are first to admit fault by saying we are sorry, and second to forgive someone who has hurt us. Our freedom from sin and pain comes when we return to our saintly Soul Self!

Chapter Twelve

CHAPTER TWELVE

FROM THE "I" TO THE "WE"

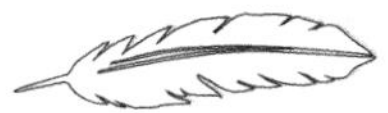

"Love is happy when it is able to give something. The ego is happy when it is able to take something."

— OSHO

The "I" is the inner ego craving attention, and the "we" is the uniting of souls. When we focus on the "I," we can become isolated and feel alone. Those feelings spark emotions, and we question God.

Staying in alignment with our Soul Self may seem like a full-time job. Taking time to meditate, heal, forgive, shift our thoughts from fear to love, change our diet, release old behaviors and the like can and will require time to assimilate into our life. A healthy life is a balanced life. What happens to a lot of people when they dive into healing their life is that they begin to isolate themselves from outside influences. In the beginning this can be supportive, but as time goes on, the isolation becomes a barrier that divides the "I" from the "we."

Katie, whom you met in chapter one, came for a healing session on a warm and sunny summer day. This session was for her, not her son Braedyn;

she had been ill for a couple of years and was feeling completely depleted. As we began her session, the Angels spoke about Katie's empathic gifts. When I asked if she knew that she had this gift, Katie replied with a "Yes." I was shown that while Katie had knowledge of her gift, she wasn't aware of how to manage it within her everyday life.

The Angels moved on to the relationships that challenged Katie. Not only were they difficult in nature, but she was also dealing with unresolved pain. This pain was manifesting in her body through the illness she had acquired because her energetic system was worn down with the pains of the past. Although Katie is gifted in her connection and had been diligent about the time she spent on doing the "you work" to connect to Spirit, she had avoided the "you work" to heal the relationships that challenged her. While she evaded facing those past memories, they kept presenting themselves to her in different circumstances.

Those old relationships were now replaying through employees taking advantage of her kind nature at her business and friends who didn't respect her. The flow of wealth was also at a standstill for Katie, as she shared her gifts freely yet received little in return for the work she put forth. And though she was hurt by both of these situations and focused on how to resolve them, they were actually teaching her to heal past wounds and invite healthier relationships, energy, and wealth into her life.

Katie's escaping the past was actually a form of manipulating the energy in which she lived. She controlled the energy of the past by not speaking or looking at the painful relationships with an open heart and mind. Rather, Katie was pushing those feelings and emotions down, and this had her living in victimhood. Avoiding the act of forgiving those who caused her pain was inviting still more pain to enter her being. I gently explained how this energy turns to manipulation and informed her that such manipulation is a telltale sign of empathic gifts.

By Katie avoiding the people who challenged her, she was in a sense protesting learning how their energy was reflecting a lesson for her. Katie was choosing to avoid her healing and creating healthy boundaries for these challenging relationships. Her body became worn down by the energetic guilt and anger, and this kept her living in pain.

The Angels say this is a big reveal of how we focus on serving the "I," which is our ego's needs, wants, and desires. We tend to walk away or close off those painful relationships to protect our "I." This is a way to avoid the valuable lesson being presented to us and heal the "we," which is who we are in this life and our connection to love. There are always two sides to a relationship, and regardless of how we've been hurt, we still have our own work to do.

While Katie and I discussed how spending time on working with Spirit was a good point of focus for her "I," we also spoke about how forgiving would release the energy she had inadvertently stored in her body and would be for the greater good of the "we." Katie left the session with Spirit's guidance around specific foods to introduce into her diet and a set of "you work" exercises to alleviate the pain in her body.

This particular session offered me a good opportunity to explain what the Angels have taught me about energy: energy between people and situations looks like threads of light, similar to a Twizzlers Pull 'n' Peel. These thin cords connect us to the world around us. While we may be unaware that these cords are there, we definitely can feel when our energy is being drained from us. In order to stop being depleted, we can cut the energetic connection. We can separate from the relationships that don't serve us in a healthy way by following the Twizzler meditation. This allows us to heal the "we" by focusing on love for both points of view. This practice will help us welcome new, loving, and vibrant relationships into our life. We heal because we can face the painful lesson and release the suffering.

Exercise

Following the same theory, I teach my clients and students this powerful healing method of release as a meditation.

Twizzler Meditation:

Set yourself up in your meditative spot with your journal at your side.

Say a prayer with intent, such as: "Dear God, please surround me with Your pure, loving energy. Help me to be open to see and know what is draining my energy or not serving me. Amen."

Begin by sitting with your spine straight and cycle breathe several times. Allow your body to release any tension or stress.

Place the palms of your hands over your heart center. Allow this to help you feel safe and protected, with God's love surrounding you in a shimmering white light.

Bring your attention to the center of your chest. Allow your chest to rise and fall like ocean waves do, effortlessly cascading up the sand. Feel your heart chakra begin to open with the most beautiful emerald-green light that encompasses your body.

Notice how your heart chakra fills the entire room you are in with healing emerald energy.

Within your heart chakra, begin to notice cords of energy. Take a moment to sense these cords and what they look like. Notice that while some of the cords look healthy and strong, others may look darker and less vibrant.

Visualize either a person or an event that has caused you pain. Just allow the shape to take form in front of you without connecting to the stories your mind wants you to replay. As this person or situation takes form, you feel safe surrounded by Divine love, and you can see the state of the cord that connects you to that which is in front of you.

With a prayerful mind, bow in reverence to this energy while inviting your energy cord to disconnect.

As your cord is released, it returns to a healthy state and is replaced in your heart. A sense of relief washes over you, and the energy of the past fades out of sight.

Your body absorbs the love, and a renewal of energy take place.

You can invite another situation or person forward, again bowing in reverence, honoring love while releasing the energy cord that binds you.

Each time you release a cord, you fill with love and hope, and the past no longer drains you.

By bowing to the pain, you honor the person and lesson even if you do not fully comprehend the why. You know just by releasing the cord connection you've gained compassion, and with that compassionate heart you and the other are set free.

Repeat this meditation when you feel drained or when the past comes knocking at your memory's back door!

Journal:

Write in your journal about how you are feeling and any experiences you had.

Shared Pain, Shared Healing

God says that we are all equal, and therefore your pain is His pain. When we hold on to the past, we forgo the miracle of healing to take place in the present moment. Each time we invite the pain of the past to leave our body with love, an energetic shift takes place for us and the person on the other end of the energy Twizzler. This is how we can change our point of view from the "I" to the "we."

CHAPTER THIRTEEN

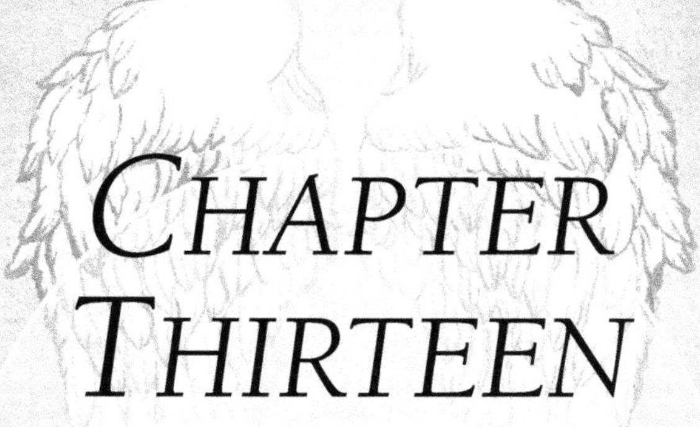

CHAPTER THIRTEEN

Love Spark

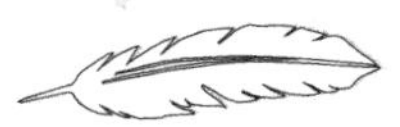

"Here is where our real selfhood is rooted, in the divine spark or seed, in the image of God imprinted on the human soul. The True Self is not our creation but God's. It is the self we are in our depths. It is our capacity for divinity and transcendence."

— SUE MONK KIDD

What I have learned through being a spiritual medium, healer, teacher, and author who channels Angels, Spirit and Divine love is that we are all capable of healing. We are equal in God's eyes, and each of us is talented and gifted. Each one of us is meant to be here. I practice my faith and do my "you work" each and every day in order to love myself, show up and serve, guide others, and follow where God leads me. Thus, I am accountable for practicing what I teach and how I live my life.

Being a loving and dedicated wife and mother have always been my main priorities, and I've added self-love to that list. What the Angels have shared with me is that if I don't self-love, I become depleted on all levels. In return for my continued efforts in choosing love first and practicing my "you work" through the meditations and exercises I've shared in this book, I am able to release pain, turn away from fear, and raise my consciousness.

We Are Love

When we connect to the Divine truth that we are love, the miracle moments that are meant for us are welcomed in through our faith. We can all practice our "you work" to show up for ourselves first, then for others. Throughout this book, I've offered reflections and tools that will repattern the old fear thought system, replacing it with a love-inspired one.

We are energetic beings. Each of us has an ego mind which likes to have a logical or idealistic explanation for attitudes, behaviors, opinions, and actions. Labeling, judging, misinterpreting, and jumping to conclusions about each other has become a norm in society. Yet if and when our thought system changes from a fear point of view to a love point of view, that love sparks in our being and we rise to our own greatness, knowing that the Divine truth of God's love guides and heals both our perceptions and our life. Then we live in an energetically balanced state of being.

As you've read again and again in this book, we all have fears. I, too, have to continually practice my "you work" so that I can teach and share Spirit's messages and be the light for others when I am called to do so. Just like you, I must pay attention to the moments when fear's tones come into the picture. I must remember that the only difference between humans and evil is love; that without love, fear can easily take over a human soul and turn it evil. It can also be turned back, though; even this can be healed, because God forgives everyone who asks and accepts His love. This moment of turn is a love spark moment!

Our Miracle Moments

Miracles are available to every soul. Yes, this means you! The gifts from the Divine are meant to help guide and support us through the good times, the challenging times, and the times we fall from grace. The Angels will always provide us with love and assistance, as long as we are open to it! We simply must remember that fear, and therefore evil, is an energy and will do what it must to rid us and the planet of love. Our choice to live with love reflects Divine love outward, healing fear.

Understanding ourselves or our loved ones on a soul level will enrich our life far beyond what our mind can show us. Basically, what I am saying here is that when we take the time to do the "you work," we are creating sparks of love that turn into a flame. Following the twelve Goddess principles, the "you work," journaling, and choosing love are the tools we need to call out those fear tones, preventing its lower energy from destroying love. When we commit to this, our lives are forever changed.

Be kind to yourself as you do your "you work," as healing takes time and energy. Don't try and go quickly; as they say, Rome wasn't built in a day, and your healing will require patience and self-love. Living in your alignment allows you to live authentically and true to your soul. Your continued practice, dedication, and openness will lead you to discover the many layers that make you who you are.

Having the courage to do the "you work" is that calling from within. We must be willing to brave our fears, our pain, and our suffering, facing them head-on with faith as our shield and God as our comfort. It's scary to face our pain. It's lonely to be brave. It's unsettling to be vulnerable. It's painful to go it alone and not know our Soul Self, but love has now sparked within and now you can choose to align with her.

Messages Heal

In sharing the messages in the previous chapters from the Angels and my clients, I've offered you a choice: you can either receive love's guidance and move toward a new way of living or deny love and continue forward in fear. We are all human, so please don't misinterpret my message; we all experience fear, and we continue to be challenged by our fear even after we choose to live in love. I encounter my Shmego guy each time I am guided to give a talk, write a book, blog or share a post on social media. I have to face the fears with which he challenges me. I have to bravely choose to either ignore fear's lies and be the light or to return to that hidden place behind my truths.

The same is true for each of us. We are living in a time that is in need of a great healing. It's time to heal our pains, our thoughts, and our actions. Love is needed to clean up our opinions. It is an era in which we are called to face our greatest fears and see beyond them to experience love fully. Love heals, while fear imprisons. When we make the choice to be the love, we can be of service and help humanity, or we can choose to join the chaos and help fear give birth to evil by spreading its propaganda. We are each responsible for our own energy. Whether we identify ourselves as an empath, sensitive soul, or even a pure of heart, the time to rise to our own occasion is upon us! If we take a stand with love, together we can raise the energy and consciousness of our planet.

My tried-and-true methods for healing fear and standing in our Soul Self, through meditation and prayer, can be found throughout this book. This final exercise is what I have found works better than any other to connect to my Soul Self.

Exercise

The Angels guided me to develop this exercise and there is a mystical experience connected to it. Each time we use this meditation, we will experience a beautiful, loving, and heightened sense of being.

Soul Self Meditation:

Begin by sitting in meditation posture on the floor with your spine straight and your legs loosely crossed. Use a meditation pillow to balance your hips so they have an equal connection to the ground.

Once you are settled, begin breathing to connect to the Earth through your root chakra.

Wrap your hands around your feet and gently massage the center of your soles with your thumbs three times in a circular motion. Then softly press your thumbs into the center of your soles.

Be still in your breathing and in your mind. Envision the crown of your head opening.

The flow of heavenly energy begins moving through your body and settles in the soles of your feet. Sense the root of who you are in this life as you notice your soul lift forward in your body, rising to the skin's surface. The heavenly energy cascades like a waterfall, embracing your being. This mystical fountain of love showers all around you as your skin absorbs the bountiful energy.

Your mind lifts to an elevated state of being as your internal vision floats upward to meet this expanded view.

The veil is open for you to experience your senses.

Your intention is to move with love and think love while being one with love.

Allow any thoughts in the mind to move to the side, making room for love's presence and enlightened tones.

Stay in this moment as long as you need.

When you're ready, slowly move your arms and legs and roll your neck from side to side before opening your eyes.

Journal:

Write in your journal about how you are feeling and any experiences you had.

Brave Is the New Sexy

As this book concludes, I want you to have the confidence and tools to spread and share love fully. I believe that our time together is not ending; rather, it's a love spark moment that will offer up limitless healing, as long as we go forward choosing love first. Remember the two universal truths that the Angels shared: One, that the soul is infinite, meaning you are here on Earth and with God at the same time. This also means that the separation we experience when a loved one dies is just of the physical body; the soul remains connected to us always. Two, we all want to be loved, equally. To express love, we must first love ourselves then share that outward with others.

Miracles happen when we follow our Goddess path, heal our fear addictions, and practice our "you work," respecting and loving ourselves. Love will guide us then to find compassion and equality in others, practice forgiveness, and offer love instead of spreading fear's propaganda. This takes extreme bravery. We're up for the challenge.

We're brave enough to see that our pain does not define us. The fastest way to experience our greatness is by finding the love that is available to us in this moment of time, honoring this love with our gratitude, and then sharing love with another. Sharing love builds relationships, character, strength, happiness, a full heart, and a joy-filled life. Calling on angelic guidance as we heal will enrich our life. Standing alone in our vulnerability as we do the "you work" can be the scariest place we've ever been, yet it is the most rewarding. Being brave to work through pain is part of our brilliance, and that is the beauty that makes us shine our sexy Soul Self!

My Prayer for You

May God bless you with the strength, courage, and vulnerability so you may be humble and whole. Be brave. Be you.

Be the love you've always wanted to receive and your life will be fulfilled. How do I know this? It's simple: Angels don't lie!

Acknowledgments

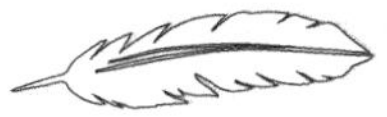

And now, I release a sigh of relief: Phew!

The truth is channeling Spirit comes with ease, but writing comes with a bit of stress, due to the challenges of being a dyslexic gal. Thankfully, with Spirit's guidance, love, and the gift of my amazing supportive team, we are blessed to come together and bring another book to life. Love, respect, and gratitude for my editor, Chandika, whose gentle wisdom and supportive energy helped shape my writing and books.

I thank God for my loving parents, Pamela and Richard, and for all the hard work and love you poured into our family! Thank you for blessing me with my siblings, Chrissy, Richie, and Paul. I love you all!

I thank God for my husband and best friend, Brian. It is through your dedication to our family and to me for the past thirty-four years that I am able to spread my wings, sharing love and helping so many people. I love you, Street 26/26, always!

I also thank God for both my birthed children and bonus ones. You are the light that brightens my life!

My daughter Lauren and her hubby, Jeff, and the three grands they have blessed us with: Riley Roo, Maisy Daisy, and oh … Henry.

My son Jason and his bride, Kara, along with the sweetest grand girls, Hadley Hoots and Reagan.

My son Casey and his wife and three children TBA ... ha!

My Molly Dolly.

I am beyond blessed to know and work with amazingly insightful and lovely souls:

Colleen, whose lifelong friendship I adore! Having you by my side through the ups and downs of life, along with your keen eye and gifted editorial skills with dyslexia, have been a saving grace in my life. I love you!

My sister by marriage Eileen, thank you for coming into this project with an open heart and willingness to share your incredible gifts and talents. Your presence in this book project and my life is a gift from God!

Casey and Kathy, with gratitude and love, I thank you both for believing in my concept of a radio show called *Angles Don't Lie* and gifting me the airtime in which to share Spirit's messages. You know, I know what I know because *Angels don't lie*!

With my heart pouring over with love, I thank each of my earthly angels and spiritual peeps whose loving wisdom and friendship I treasure: Kari, Carly, Kim, Heather, Pam, and Lana—I see you!

It is with sincerest gratitude that I thank each of my clients for the opportunity to share the loving messages the Angels send me, and especially to those clients who have offered their experiences for me to share in this book. Your bravery inspires me! Amen.

About the Author

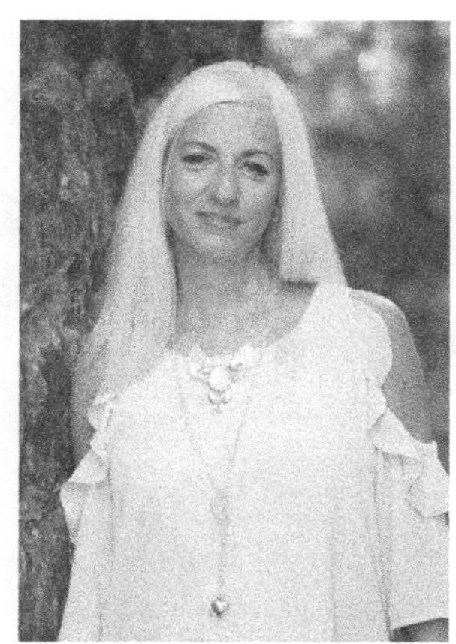

Internationally acclaimed spirital medium, healer, author and speaker, Jeanne Street, is a Catholic girl in an Angel world. She works with the Spiritual realm embodying the Holy Spirit while illuminating Divine compassion and love through her work.

Jeanne was born into this life with the beautiful gift of connection. She has the ability to see, feel, hear and speak to both the departed and celestial beings.

Through her connection and clear knowing her sessions and readings are precise and detailed. Jeanne has helped thousands of individuals navigate through difficult events in their lives. Jeanne's deepest desire is to help people heal their pain and trauma.

Jeanne provides connection to Spirit, Angels and departed loved ones through private and small group readings, large group events, and through her books, The Goddess You and The Goddess Journal, Believe . . . Angels Don't Lie and Angels Don't Lie Believe . . .Journal. She also offers Divine lifestyle products, accessories and a vast array of resources that are available on her website.

Jeanne's loving and accurate connections have transformed the lives of her private clients and public podcast listeners, as well as the live audience on her show Angels Don't Lie.

Jeanne resides in Connecticut with her devoted husband of 35 years, her 4 grown children, her daughter and son in law and 5 grandchildren and counting.

Spiritual support for your soul's growth

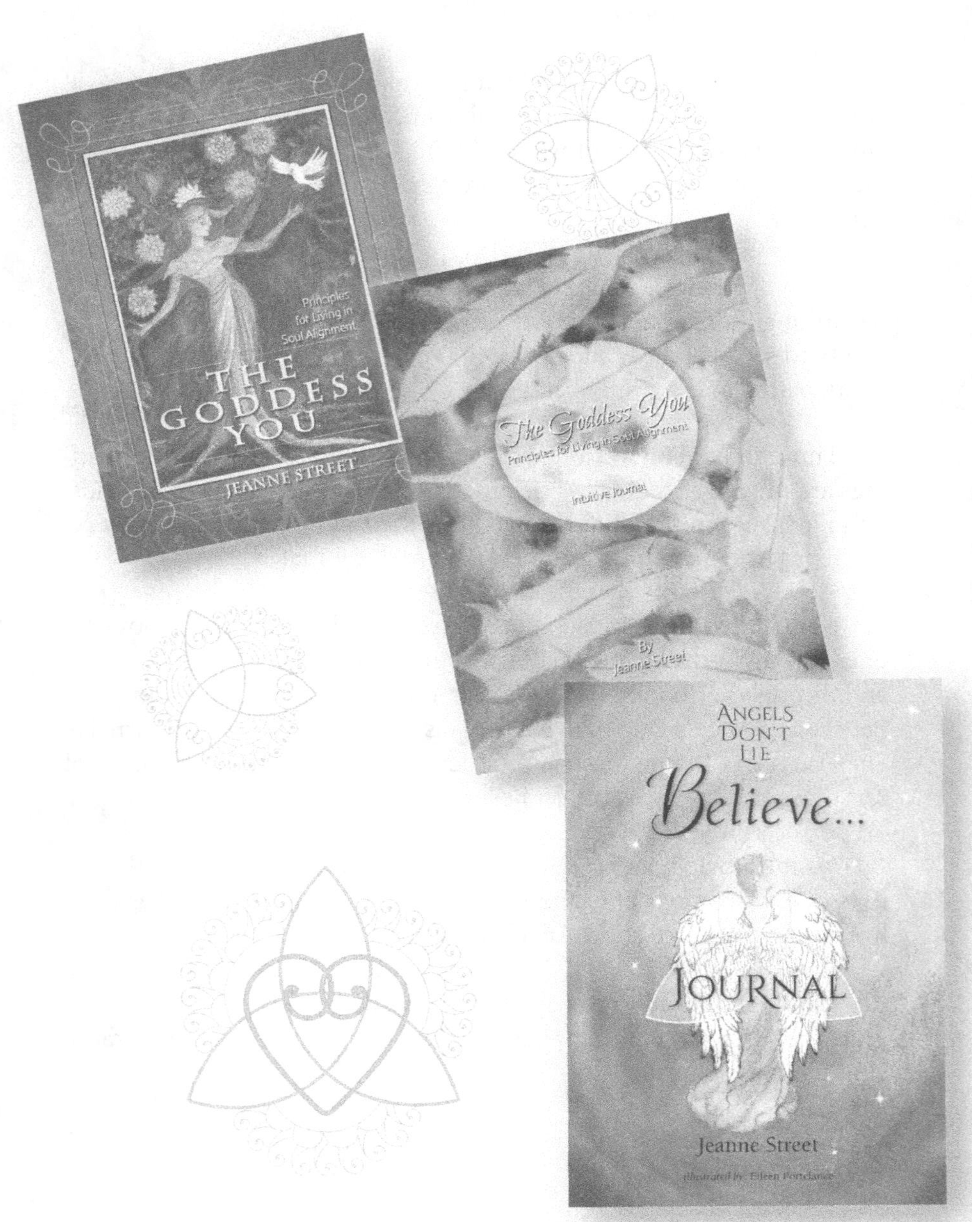

Continue to feel supported & spritually aligned EVERYDAY!

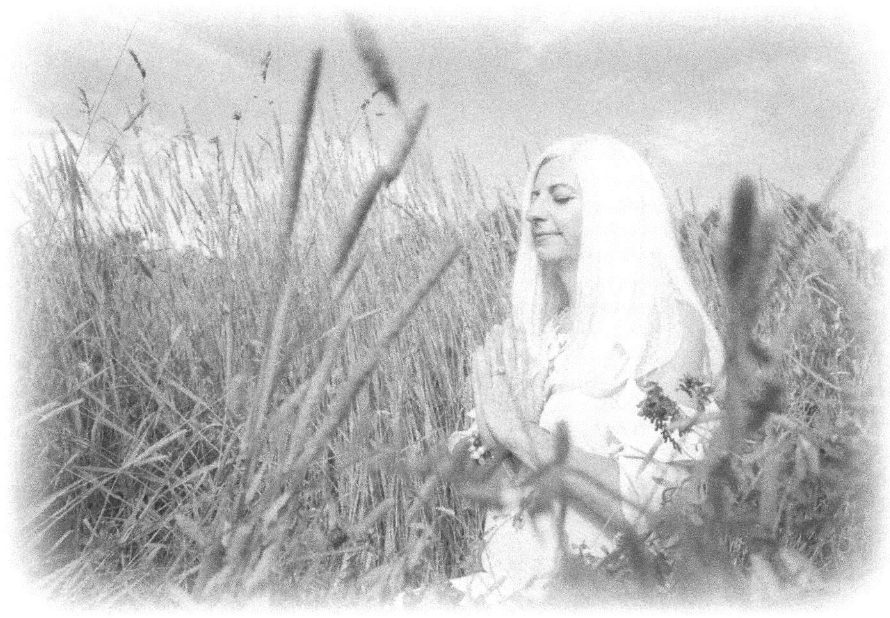

visit me at….

www.jeannestreet.com

https://www.facebook.com/Jeannestreetmedium/

https://www.instagram.com/jeannestreetmedium/

CPSIA information can be obtained
at www.ICGtesting.com
Printed in the USA
BVHW011305240720
584428BV00019B/81/J

9 780997 466669